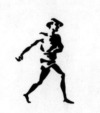

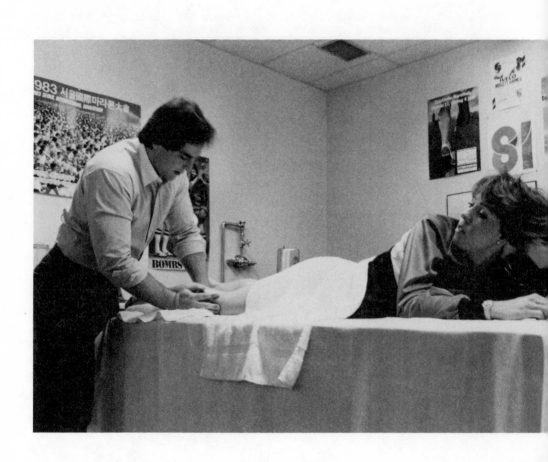

ATHLETIC MASSAGE

Rich Phaigh
and Paul Perry

Photographs by Warren Morgan

SIMON AND SCHUSTER   NEW YORK

To my mother, Louise, without whose constant encouragement and support I could not have approached this level of achievement. Thanks, Mom.

—Rich Phaigh

To my wife, Dee, an encouraging and lovely soul.

—Paul Perry

Copyright © 1984 by Rich Phaigh and Paul Perry
All rights reserved
including the right of reproduction
in whole or in part in any form
Published by Simon and Schuster
A Division of Simon & Schuster, Inc.
Simon & Schuster Building
Rockefeller Center
1230 Avenue of the Americas
New York, New York 10020
SIMON AND SCHUSTER and colophon are registered trademarks of
Simon & Schuster, Inc.
Designed by Eve Kirch
Manufactured in the United States of America

10 9 8 7 6 5 4 3 2 1

Library of Congress Cataloging in Publication Data
Phaigh, Rich.
   Athletic massage.
   1. Massage.   2. Sports—Physiological aspects
I. Perry, Paul, date.   II. Title.
RC1226.P48   1984   615.8'22   84-14177
ISBN 0-671-52565-4

Contents

Part Three
Curative Massage

Foreword

My running career has always been plagued by injuries. Since the age of eleven, when I first discovered my talent for running, I have had several battles with shin splints, calf muscle pulls, Achilles tendinitis, hamstring tears and all the other injuries that afflict runners.

Some of the more serious injuries have led to surgery. Four times I have been operated on for lower leg problems that wouldn't heal. The most recent surgery on my shins was in 1981. Due to complications caused by anti-inflammatory drugs, the recovery time from that surgery was much longer than normal. And as would be expected, any running that I did was extremely painful. I went through several types of therapy to relieve the pain: I tried acupressure, acupuncture, electrical stimulation, casts and all sorts of pain drugs. Then I met Rich Phaigh.

I saw Rich two to three times a week for 45 minute sessions of deep muscle massage. I remember that first session. Rich probed the injured area with his thumbs. He pressed so deep that I was sure he was causing more harm than good. I remember thinking that this would be just another in a long line of worthless remedies.

But it wasn't. It turned out to be the remedy that worked. Seven months after surgery, I was able to train normally.

The positive effects of massage were evident immediately after I resumed training. Soreness didn't linger, nor did the tightness that used to stay with me after training runs. Instead, Rich's frequent massages kept my muscles loose and free of the body chemicals of exertion that had previously affected my performance.

7

My training runs became painless, with fewer injuries than in the past. And with my shorter recovery time, I soon began training at a consistently high level, better than ever before.

The rest is history. Since discovering massage I have set eight world records, won several national titles and been able to win two world championship titles. I am in the best shape of my life due to my lack of injury.

I owe most of my high fitness level to Rich and his method of athletic massage. I know this is true because I don't get Rich's massage treatments when I travel for an extended period of time. Then, old injuries creep back and recovery time increases with each hard run. When that happens I know it's time to get back to Rich's massage table.

I recommend massage to athletes at any level of ability, from world class to the weekend competitor. It will not only improve your performance, it will speed your recovery time and cut down on the number of muscle injuries. And all of that will make any sport more fun, which is really what it's all about anyway.

—MARY DECKER

PART ONE

MASSAGE IS THE MESSAGE

1 · INTRODUCTION

In 1983, a journalist was in Eugene, Oregon, doing one of those "week-in-the-life" stories on Mary Decker that graced so many magazines that year. He had followed her in a van as she did a long run on Saturday ("I had to ride in a vehicle," he explained. "There's no way I could *run* with her!"), gone to lunch at a fine local restaurant ("that's one thing I *can* do with her") and visited her coach ("he is *definitely* there to keep her from running herself into the ground").

By the time they showed up at my therapy room at the Athletics West Track Club, Mary was edgy. She had run a hard thirty to forty miles so far that week and was sore all over. On top of that, she had some areas of specific soreness in one of her calves.

"I think she is out of it for the rest of the week," said the journalist, receiving an immediate cold stare from Mary for his opinion.

I went to work. I massaged her shoulders first, eliminating the stress that had built up from the swinging of her arms. I worked down her spine, attacking the knots that had settled in from the relentless pounding of running. Finally, I worked on the legs—the tight hamstrings, the tired Achilles tendons and the particularly sore calf. She grimaced as I probed the calf, and so did the journalist, who wrote furiously in his notebook throughout the massage.

When the treatment was over, Mary pushed herself up from the padded table and walked slowly to the dressing room. Later that day, she was back on the road, running as though the soreness had never hampered her.

The journalist was impressed.

A couple of days later, he came back, armed with his notebook, which was full of glowing comments from Mary about the powers of massage. "I didn't make any progress as a runner until Rich started working on my legs," was one of the things she said. "The massage hurt for a while, but I wouldn't have made such a strong comeback from injury without him."

Mary's coach went even further. "For the past two years, Mary has remained relatively healthy," said the usually reserved Dick Brown. "If Rich had not been there when she needed him, Mary would not have run so well, if at all."

She called what I was doing to her legs "magic" and claimed that it was perhaps the single most important factor in her success.

The journalist wanted to know more about me and about massage. His notebook contained several questions that he had penned during her therapy and the interviews afterward. It would only take a minute, he said, and began asking questions.

I hadn't been expecting him, so the answers to his questions, which were published in the magazine for which he worked, were much less technical than I would have liked. Here are more complete answers to those questions.

Why does an athlete need massage?

Exercise is good for us. We all know this is true. Exercise provides healthy stress by elevating the heart rate, increasing blood flow to the skin, injecting tissues with oxygen, increasing the size and efficiency of the heart and lungs and releasing a variety of chemicals in the brain that makes us feel better than before exertion.

Now the bad news: exercise stresses and strains the muscle tissues. It also can injure the tendons and ligaments, which are frequently stretched beyond their normal bounds by the athlete's enthusiasm or the demands of the sport. Exercise also tears the fibers, stretches the fascia (the clear, tough covering of the muscle) and accounts for blood and fluid build-up which leaves the exercised muscle stiff and sore.

So what does massage do?

Massage reaches these exercise-damaged muscles. Done properly, the deep and educated probing stimulates circulation, increases lymphatic flow, breaks up fibrosis that binds one muscle fiber to another, relaxes muscle spasms and relieves pain. All without drugs. All without expensive medical equipment. All with just oil and your properly used hands.

Why does massage work?

Let's start with lymph. Thick and colorless, lymph is the lubricating fluid of the muscles, the motor oil of the human body. Not only does it decrease friction between the muscles, it aids in the removal of lactic acid, that painful by-product of exertion that causes muscles to sting. It also helps to remove other harmful chemical by-products of exertion from the muscles.

Lymph is produced by a series of almond-sized glands located at several points on the body. The lymphatic system has no pump. Lymph is excreted into the tissues and circulates by osmosis, gravity, muscular contractions or massage.

The only thing that stimulates lymphatic flow better than massage is exercise. But the problem with exercise is that it creates waste products that need to be floated away by lymph.

Massage increase the effectiveness of blood circulation. Superficial massage—like the Swedish method—does little more than change skin temperature, but deep massage increases blood flow. One scientific study showed that ten minutes of deep stroking and kneading of a calf doubled the blood flow to that area for more than forty minutes. Ten minutes of exercise, on the other hand, increased (not doubled) the blood flow for only ten minutes.

Of course, exercise pumps considerable blood and oxygen to the muscles, encouraging the exchange of oxygen-filled blood for carbon dioxide–filled blood. But it also increases the amount of waste that needs to be removed. All of this is a vicious circle that leads to muscle soreness. Massage breaks that circle. It flushes the tissues with blood without creating the by-products that accompany exercise.

And then, of course, there's fibrosis.

What is fibrosis?

I thought you would never ask. After exercise, you have probably experienced general soreness or a tightening of a certain area. Maybe you have run your fingers over a sore muscle and thought it felt swollen or lumpy. Perhaps "knotted" was the word you used. Well, that knotting is called spasm, and it occurs when fatigued muscle fibers tangle and remain contracted.

Fibrosis is likely to occur at the ends of muscles, where the fibers aren't used so much and therefore have less elasticity. They aren't in as good shape as the rest of the muscle. It can be caused by fatigue, when the fibers run out of glycogen and the build-up of the chemicals of exercise keeps them from working. It can also be caused by torn fibers that heal improperly and don't get the nourishment they need.

In either case the fibers protect themselves by twisting around each other like wound-up rubber bands. And like just such a rubber band, fibrosis has a way of spreading, moving up the muscle fiber until the muscle is seriously shortened. This is when pulls and tears can happen—sometimes with just normal use.

Wouldn't stretching be just as helpful as massage in the case of spasm?

A good stretching routine will pull some of the knots out, but it can't match the powers of massage for spreading and soothing the fatigued strands of muscle. Deep massage, using the strokes shown in the next chapter, separates the fibers from one another, stretching the muscle across its breadth in a way that nothing else can.

Massage isn't a cure-all. It can't make a person run faster, although one masseur has claimed it can improve a runner's performance by 20 percent. It does, however, perform seven functions:

1. it prevents muscle and tendon injuries;
2. it reduces the strain and discomfort of training;
3. it eliminates the ups and downs normally found in training;
4. it helps cure chronic injuries;
5. it helps heal acute injuries properly so the injured areas do not become a source of continued trouble;
6. it restores lost mobility;
7. it stops muscle spasms to restore normal muscular functions.

What sport is massage good for?

Any sport at all. Although it can't in itself improve performance, it can restore the body to a state in which everything is working properly.

Obviously there are some sports that require massage more than others. Those who practice strenuous sports—and in particular sports that require strenuous training—will garner more benefit from massage than those who engage in nonstrenuous sports, for obvious reasons. The former are the people whom I see in my capacity as staff masseur for Athletics West. Without frequent massage, the runners and other athletes who come there would have a very high frequency of injury.

You said massage is good for any athlete. Come on, golfers, too?

Sure—golfers, tennis players, handball players, participants in any kind of sport that requires you to be fine-tuned to perform at your best. Chess players and fishermen are about the only sportsmen I can think of who wouldn't be helped by massage.

There are many golfers who benefit from massage. Golf, like any other sport, requires a perfectly synchronized chain of muscular contractions. If one of these contractions is even slightly out of kilter, it can affect the accuracy with which a golfer hits the ball in the same way that a club that is slightly warped would affect a golfer's game.

As you might expect, some football players are strong proponents of massage. Jim Nance of the New England Patriots found massage so important that he had trainer Jack Meagher perform it during the game. That's right, during the fourth quarter Meagher was out there working on Nance's legs. Nance always said that his legs were dead by then, and the massage put spring back into the muscles.

Why didn't he use electric stimulation like so many other football players?

Because electric stimulation mimics the normal expansion and contraction of the muscle. It uses a little power pack that hooks up to the muscles and literally makes them work. That's the problem with it: making them work causes a build-up of the by-products of exhaustion. It doesn't eliminate spasms, break up fibrosis or flush toxic waste. Electric stimulation should be used to rehabilitate and strengthen a muscle that can't be exercised normally.

So why don't more athletes use massage?

For members of a football team, for example, the number of team members alone makes it impossible for the trainer to massage all of them. A professional team has forty-five players. A college team has even more. A trainer doesn't have enough time to massage all of them, especially if he wants to use preventive massage, which should be done a couple of times per week.

Amateur athletics don't get massaged because they can't afford the expense. If you were to pay to get your legs massaged twice a week, the cost would be at least sixty dollars per month. And even if you were getting massaged, you might not be getting the type of massage that is best for an athlete. The type of massage I do is a combination of friction massage, which has its origins in Germany, and Swedish massage. By using strokes from these two schools, I have combined the movements that best improve circulation to a muscle to remove its knots and soothe its aches.

I'm so convinced that active people can be helped by massage that I agreed immediately to write this book when the idea was first suggested to me. Mary Decker, too, was enthusiastic. Alberto Salazar liked the idea so much that, like Mary, he agreed to pose for some of the photos. "Massage is one of the basics of training that somehow got lost," he said. "I know that without it, I would be injured much more than I am now."

That is why we all came together to do this book. I have drawn on more than twelve years of experience as an athletic masseur, and with the help of Mary, Alberto, and Margaret Groos, I'm showing you how to put that knowledge to good use.

2 · THE MAGIC OF MASSAGE

The resurgence of athletic massage is due to its rediscovery by runners. Many of them saw—as I did—Lasse Viren's incredible performance in the 1972 Olympics. The Finnish runner was able to compete in two of the Olympiad's most difficult events, the 5,000-meter and 10,000-meter runs, winning both.

Aside from being in remarkable condition, Viren's secret was daily massage—deep massage (some say painfully deep massage that may have inured him to the agony of running so many fast miles in so few days).

When runners saw Viren's success, they wanted to copy everything about "the Flying Finn." And one thing they copied right away was massage.

Nineteen seventy-two was the first year that I practiced massage professionally. Following the Olympics of that year, the demand for massage increased dramatically among distance runners. Unfortunately, the cost was prohibitive for most athletes, who at the time were amateurs in the truest sense and could not afford massage on a regular basis.

In 1977, the Nike shoe company founded the Athletics West Track Club in Eugene, Oregon, and hired Ilopo Nikkoli, a Finnish masseur who was nicknamed "Deep Thumbs" by the athletes because of his extremely deep strokes.

His work was met with skepticism by some, particularly since it was so painful. But as the runners experienced fewer injuries due to his work, the popularity of massage increased.

When Ilopo left the track club to return to Finland, I was hired to replace him.

Since I am not as heavy with the thumbs as my predecessor, the athletes don't call me "Deep Thumbs." A few call me "Magic Fingers," because of the magic they think that my fingers work. But it isn't magic. What I do is just massage.

Like running, skiing or a walk around the block, massage feels good. And like all those forms of exercise, massage is good for us. Friction massage rolls and stretches muscles in a way that nothing can imitate. It produces increased blood flow, or hyperemia, through capillary dilation, an expansion of the blood-carrying capillary vessels that improves circulation and milks waste products from tissues. It also helps to break up scar tissue, which when left untreated can be as irritating to a muscle as a grain of sand in the eye.

Massage loosens muscle fibers, separating them from one another so they can act freely, with more flexibility. It also helps lengthen muscles shortened by the frequent and hard contractions of athletics. It eliminates fatigue, promotes relaxation, relieves swelling, reduces muscle tension and helps prevent soreness. It can even speed recovery from injury.

Sounds too good to be true? Let's take a brief look at the physiology of massage to see how it does all this.

Circulation

Numerous medical studies have proven the value of massage in improving blood circulation in the capillaries as well as in the veins and arteries.

One researcher who observed the massage process by microscopic means saw that light pressure on muscle fibers produces an instantaneous—although temporary—dilation of the capillaries, which in turn improves circulation to tissue. He also found that the capillaries stayed open for a longer period of time when more pressure was administered.

You can make a similar observation externally by examining a massaged area several minutes (as many as forty-five, if massaged properly) after treatment. There is a flushed appearance to the skin from the blood that is drawn to the spot. That glow, and the warmth that accompanies it, is due to increased circulation caused by the massage. It is the direct result of the increase in diameter of capillary blood vessels and the resultant delivery of more blood.

Improved circulation removes waste products of exercise at a faster rate. Lactic acid, an exercise pollutant that builds up in the muscles when there is lack of oxygen, is quickly pushed out of the muscles by oxygenated blood.

This rapid removal of waste products and the oxygenation of tissue allow us to overcome fatigue or injury. Observation has shown me that this is true. Many of the athletes I treat are frequently fatigued from hard workouts. Others are injured by them. I have seen massage give speedy recovery—sometimes in just a matter of hours—mainly because of improved circulation.

But it isn't blood circulation alone that contributes to the maintenance of muscle. Lymph is a very important fluid in the lubrication and "cleaning" of our muscles.

Lymph is a watery fluid that is similar in appearance to blood plasma. It is made in lymph glands, which are located at several points on the body, usually just under the skin. They are about the size of almonds, and are constantly providing a supply of colorless corpuscles to the blood. These corpuscles help remove the chemicals of exercise from the muscles via the bloodstream, where they are eventually filtered through the kidneys and excreted.

There are many medical studies that prove the value of massage in moving large quantities of lymph fluid through the body, including some that show massage is the best treatment for chronic inflammation caused by the binding together of tissue known as fibrosis.

Fibrosis

Fibrosis is a condition in which the muscle fibers can no longer function normally. In athletes, fibrosis is a by-product of tissue injury. When tissue is torn, there is always scar formation between the fibers. This scar formation can sometimes bind muscle fibers together in such a way as to diminish or eliminate normal movement. Each fiber must be allowed to function independently for a muscle to reach full power and have total mobility. Fibrosis usually results in spasm, which is the tightening of muscle fibers to protect an injured area.

Although spasm is a protective contraction, it also reduces the blood flow to an area, which in turn reduces the flow of oxygen and nutrients and prevents the area from casting off waste products. If a spasm is severe, it has a way of wringing blood and fluid out of surrounding tissues, causing the spasm to spread even further in a muscle. Massage can increase the blood flow to an area in need. Deep strokes and cross-fiber strokes will spread the tissue, smoothing out the knots that occur in those threadlike fibers and undoing the harmful effects of fibrosis. Kneading and jostling will relax the tense area.

Scar Tissue

Sometimes a muscle shortened by spasm becomes torn. In fact, even a perfectly healthy muscle can be stretched beyond its range of motion, and a tear in the fiber or the fascia (the thin, clear membrane that covers muscle) can result.

Since damaged muscle tissue doesn't regenerate, the healing cells are of a different quality from the surrounding ones. They are strong and pliable yet somewhat irritating to the surrounding tissue.

Most people can live with this minor irritation, but for athletes, who often stress their muscles to a greater degree than nonathletes, that scar becomes a source of discomfort, creating a cycle of pain, spasm and swelling that can only be alleviated by rest, and then not entirely eliminated.

For many years, physiologists erroneously thought that massage treatment led to the absorption of scar tissue by the body. Recently, they have discovered what really happens, and the truth is even more fascinating.

Repeated deep massage aligns the cells of the scar tissue with the surrounding area. It gets rid of the rough edges of scar tissue by weaving the torn fibers back together. This eliminates the pain-causing irritation process that takes place when scar tissue comes into contact with healthy tissue.

Massage will also break adhesions formed between the scar and other muscles and will create fluid circulation inside the scar tissue to keep it soft.

The result of this is improved muscle movement, a decrease in muscle tension and, of course, more enjoyable training.

And, of Course, Relaxation

Exercise is stress. It is healthy stress in that it relieves the tensions that build up in day-to-day living, but it is still stress. And too much stress from exercise creates reactions similar to those caused by job stress: edginess, listlessness, fatigue. The common terminology for this is "overwork syndrome." Of course, a finely tuned athlete takes longer to become fatigued. And because of his higher fitness level, he comes out of it sooner than a beginning athlete. But why should he allow himself to go into this state of fatigue at all?

Although massage can't eliminate fatigue entirely—especially in athletes who train consistently hard—it can greatly reduce the chances of succumbing to the overwork syndrome.

There is no finer example of the rejuvenative powers of massage than Alberto Salazar before his world-record run in the 1982 New York City marathon. "My legs are dead," he declared one afternoon when he came in for a massage. He was going to cancel his eleven-mile evening run, but after thirty minutes of deep tissue massage, he reversed his decision and ran what was, in his words, "a fantastic workout."

There are some problems that massage has no effects upon: improper alignment of the spine, weaknesses in opposing muscle groups (hamstrings and thigh muscles, for instance), bad foot plant, improper warm-up, lack of proper conditioning, nutritional deficiencies and of course, training too heavily.

The real physiological power of massage comes from the rapid and fresh fluid exchange that it causes and its ability to realign muscles that are shortened from use or in a state of spasm from overuse.

Massage won't make the athlete stronger, but it will improve the condition of his muscles so they can work to their full potential. *Massage won't eliminate scar tissue,* but it will soften it, making it something the athlete can train with instead of fight against. *Massage won't eliminate fatigue,* but it will decrease the chances of succumbing to overwork syndrome. Although it can go a long way in eliminating fatigue, the only thing that can eliminate it entirely is common-sense training, which doesn't come from the masseur's hands.

Although massage will not increase strength or endurance, it can offer the athlete a real opportunity to reach athletic potential by allowing him to do more work.

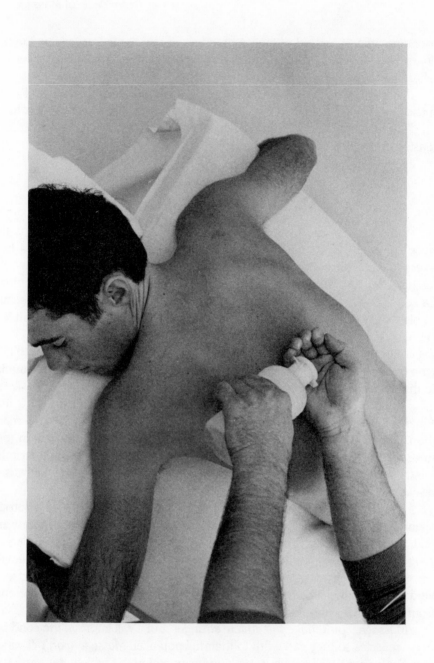

3 · METHODS OF MASSAGE

For the masseur—like the surgeon—touch is a form of sight. His hands probe the muscles, working out soreness with a variety of movements. And just like a surgeon, a masseur must know how to use his hands to be effective.

"The fingers of a good rubber will descend upon an excited and painful nerve as gently as the dew on the grass," said nineteenth-century philosopher-physician Samuel Beveridge.

Over the years my hands have become strong enough to perform thirty half-hour massages a day. That is quite a difference from the two I could perform in the beginning. You, too, may only be able to manage one or two massages, and you may need two hands where I normally use one. In time you will grow stronger and surer with your hands.

In this chapter I'll show you the movements of proper massage, including a method to compensate for lack of hand strength and stamina. But first, let's begin with the simple—but important—catalog of equipment necessary to accomplish the art of athletic massage.

Firm Surface, Oil and Confidence

The table I use is a wooden one that I made when I began studying massage. It is about four feet high and has a firm foam pad covering its entire length. At one end is a retractable headrest that is open in the center and raises even with the foam surface so the athlete can lie face down comfortably without propping his head on folded forearms to breathe.

I designed this table to accommodate the more than 3,000 massages I do each year. You can do the same, or you can buy one of the portable varieties on the market that fold up into the size of a suitcase for convenient storage.

Or you can do what most people do: use the floor. If you have a hardwood floor you will want to put down a piece of foam to cushion the athlete against the hardness and insulate him from the cold.

Even if you are on carpet, it will be necessary to cover the area beneath the person being massaged with towels or sheets. After all, we are using oil to decrease the friction between the massaging hands and the massaged muscles, and the last thing you want is an oily outline on the carpet.

What kind of oil do you use? There are some expensive massage oils available in health food stores, many of which are scented. My favorite one is a mixture of sweet almond oil, walnut oil, cocoa butter and vitamin E, which costs about fifteen dollars per gallon. Other commonly used lubricants are olive oil, peanut oil, coconut oil and even some fine powders, for those who prefer a rougher massage. Even ordinary vegetable oil works just fine. The key is to apply just enough to allow the hands to move freely over the muscles, but not so much that you can't firmly grasp the skin and keep it under control.

As important as the equipment is the athlete's comfort. Is the room warm enough? Is the floor padded enough to be comfortable? Does the athlete feel comfortable with you in your role as practitioner? Unless the answer to these questions is "yes," the athlete will not attain the deep relaxation necessary for successful massage. The purpose of athletic massage is to create a prolonged state of reduced muscle tension, increased blood and lymph circulation and a deep level of relaxation. The athlete should be relaxed going into the massage in order to be relaxed coming out of it.

One problem that frequently arises has to do with clothing. Nudity isn't mandatory in massage. Although it allows the masseur to make direct contact with the skin, if the athlete doesn't feel comfortable nude—particularly if he doesn't know his masseur well—then he can wear clothing. I recommend a backless swimsuit for women, or one with a bikini-type top. It is almost mandatory to have the legs bare, but if that is all you want uncovered, then shorts will be sufficient.

If there are problems in comfort or communication, they should be dealt with before the massage begins, to make sure the entire massage time is spent in relaxation.

The Movements and Their Meaning

I use several movements, or "strokes," designed to stretch both the length and breadth of each muscle fiber as well as encourage deep and long-term fluid flow.

The movements I use in athletic massage come from various schools. The deep strokes, for instance, are a lighter form of rolfing, a type of massage known for its painfully hard and deep treatments. Kneading, which is the same movement that is used in kneading dough, is from Swedish massage, which encourages a state of deep muscle relaxation.

I have mixed these movements and others from various disciplines to create a unique form of athletic massage.

One movement I don't use that you may be familiar with is "tapotement," those rapid, loose-fingered judo chops that boxers in old movies are always getting from their masseurs. The purpose of the movement is to enhance blood flow and relax the muscles in the treated areas, according to the practitioners of Swedish massage, who use this particular movement. I find the movement useless. Although it increases superficial circulation and general relaxation, it does little to break up fibrosis and actually has a tendency to tighten the area being treated.

I prefer to use jostling, which offers the same vibrating action as tapotement without the slapping action that tightens the muscles. A description of jostling is offered later in this chapter.

Practice these strokes carefully. Muscle is tough and probably cannot be injured by using too much pressure. But massage that is too deep can quickly become painful. Take it easy.

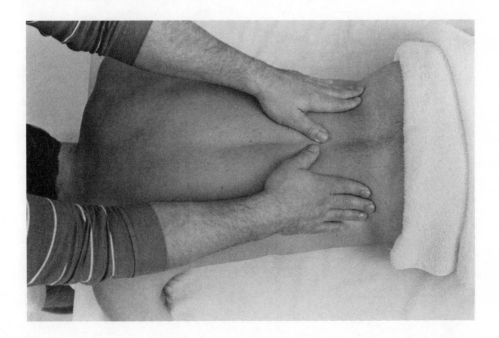

Light Stroking

Usually done with the palms of the hands, light stroking is used to apply the oils and soothe the muscles. These strokes are performed toward the heart to enhance the blood's circulation. On small regions, one hand may follow the other. On large regions, the hands may move side by side, as in the photo. But no matter how you are doing it, it is important to maintain contact with the athlete's skin. Breaking contact may cause the athlete to break his state of relaxation.

The purpose of this stroke is to apply the oil and soothe the muscles, which is why it is done first. If you start the stroke at the portion of the muscle farthest from the heart and cover the area several times, applying a little more pressure with each pass, the athlete will be properly warmed up, relaxed, and ready for the deeper strokes.

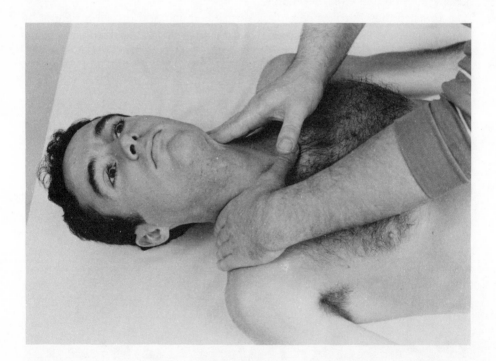

Petrissage

On areas too difficult to light-stroke with the palm of your hand, use petrissage. This is a massage movement applied in a circular motion with your fingertips. It is most often used on the neck, where the palm is too large to reach the muscles effectively, or on areas like the chest, where the smaller muscles are better served by a more directly applied light stroke.

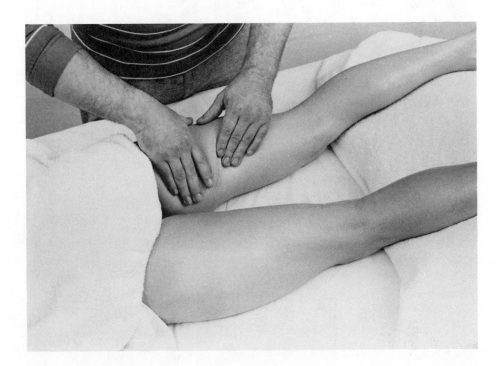

Kneading

We call this the breadmaker's stroke, because it is performed in much the same fashion as the kneading of dough. This movement is simply a matter of gently grasping a group of muscles between the thumb and fingers and, with alternating hands, squeezing the thumb and fingers together while working the muscles up and down.

Kneading is useful in assessing the state of the muscles. You can identify tension in the muscle by how difficult it is to lift and move it compared with neighboring muscles. Sometimes, when the massage is finished, it helps to go back and knead a problem area a second time. Generally the muscle will be more pliable, less likely to feel stiff or snap back.

Some masseurs believe that kneading is more effective than deep stroking in creating deep circulation and aiding in absorption of exercise by-products. I don't agree with that. I think deep strokes have a more sustained effect upon deep muscle problems than kneading, simply because they reach them better and more directly. But kneading certainly removes waste fluids from the muscles and can be a nice break from the deep strokes.

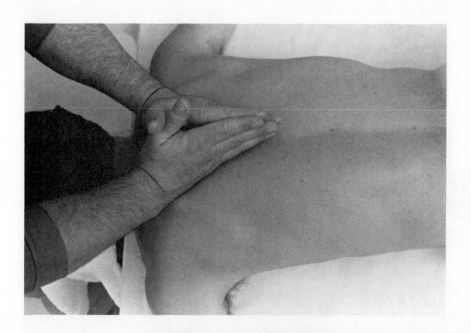

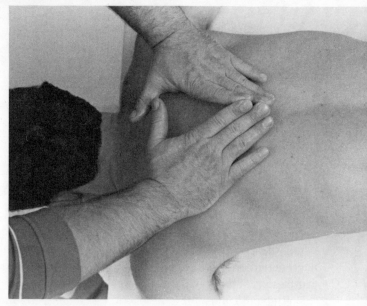

Fanning

I call this the prayer movement because it begins with the hands together in prayer fashion before they spread out to cover muscle by moving away from a central point and out to the edges of the body.

This is a movement reserved for those places on the body where muscle radiates from the body's centerline. The spine is one such place, as are the chest and abdomen. Fanning provides equal pull and pressure to take the kinks out of the muscle and improve circulation.

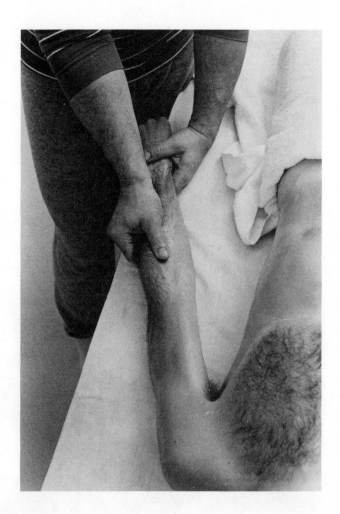

Broad Cross-Fiber Strokes

Administered with the thumb, these strokes cross the muscle at ninety-degree angles. This is one of the slow strokes, since an entire muscle has to be covered by this movement that repeatedly inches its way across muscles as the hand moves up toward the heart.

But as slow as it is, it is also one of the most valuable strokes, because it stretches the muscle across its breadth, separating fibers from one another and expanding the size of the balloonlike sheath that covers the muscle.

Only one or two muscle groups should be worked on at one time. That way you can accurately detect the problem muscles by the way they snap back instead of easily rolling over to the next muscle. By the way, when you find a problem muscle, concentrate on it by repeating this stroke several times, following with the jostling movement and then deep strokes. Repeat the process several times.

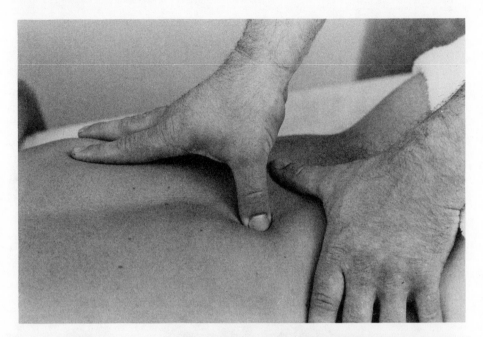

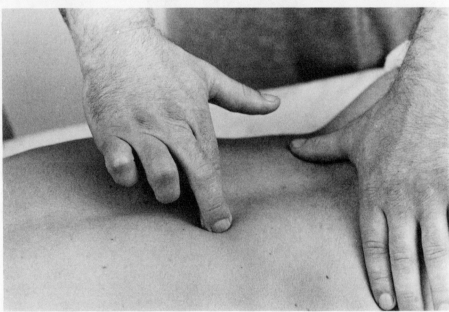

Local Cross-Fiber Strokes

Apply these strokes with the thumb or the fingertips. Although they are the most time-consuming and tiring of all the strokes, they are used only on problem areas and are therefore used less frequently than the other movements.

Problem areas in the muscle usually feel hard. When you find such a spot, work on it gently but deeply. This is accomplished by stroking the area lightly at first, pressing hard with each pass until the tightness is gone.

Local cross-fiber strokes may cause some soreness that will last a day or two, but that is normal. When injured muscles heal, scar tissue forms around them, irritating the surrounding muscles and causing pain, inflammation, spasm and the likelihood of reinjury.

Local cross-fiber strokes loosen the scar tissue, making it more pliable by pushing blood and fluid through the tissue itself.

This stroke also keeps tendons from becoming bound to their surrounding sheaths and, as do all the strokes, improves deep circulation and the elimination of wastes.

Although this stroke is effective during the rehabilitation period of muscular or connective tissue injury, it is likely to do more damage than good on a newly injured area. It should be avoided until inflammation subsides. For more about this stroke, see Chapter 13.

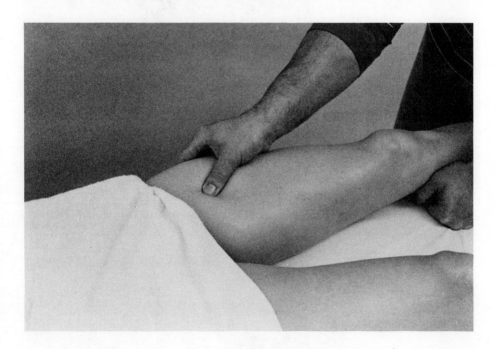

Jostling

In this stroke, you loosely grasp the muscle at the point of origin (the part closest the heart) and shake it gently back and forth while telling the athlete to relax. Repeat this as you move all the way down the muscle to the point of insertion (the part farthest from the heart). Then stroke back to the point of origin.

Jostling relaxes the athlete between rounds of deep stroking. The gentle shaking of the muscles breaks down the protective reflex response, the natural tendency to tighten a muscle when touched. A couple of passes over a tight area should relax it sufficiently.

Relaxation is important. If an athlete tightens muscles in response to your stroking, the muscle tightens inside its sheath. Instead of the affected tissue, the sheath then receives the bulk of the massage. It is relaxation that makes jostling a movement of such therapeutic value.

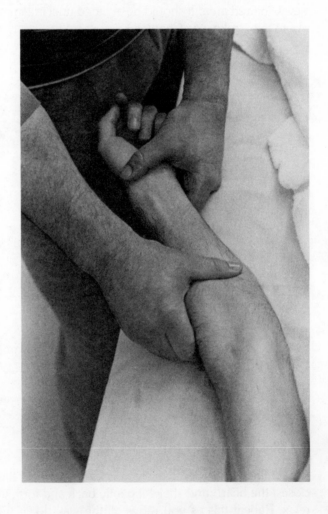

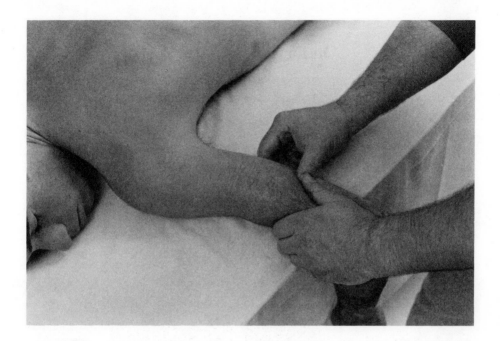

Deep Stroking

Deep stroking (shown opposite and above) is done with the pads of the thumbs, which may be held side by side, one behind the other or—in the case of beginners—one on top of the other for added strength. These movements should move the length of the muscle, beginning farthest away from the heart and moving toward it.

The deep stroke can be painful. It can also cause the athlete to tense up. If that happens, lighten up on the pressure and tell the athlete to relax. If he remains tense, jostle the area.

Hippocrates said that hard massage makes hard muscle, a statement that modern science has proven wrong. What deep stroking will do is move tremendous amounts of lymph and blood through the muscles. Hence, this stroke can greatly reduce inflammation of muscles due to fluid build-up. Because of this, I sometimes perform massages using only a light variation of deep strokes for athletes who are competing on consecutive days.

It is important, however, not to apply more pressure than is comfortable to a newly injured area, since the added longitudinal pressure can tear the muscle fibers even further.

On Developing Touch

It takes time to perform these techniques correctly. Reading about the proper methods of massage won't make you a masseur. Only "on-the-body" experience can do that.

Practice these techniques, and expect to administer a few massages that are more experimental than effective. Begin all movements gently, never applying more pressure than the athlete can comfortably tolerate. If he says it hurts, believe him and decrease intensity.

This applies especially to problem areas like knots in the muscles or "sore spots" that the athlete identifies. Work those areas with caution, listening with your ears rather than relying on your hands alone.

PART TWO

PREVENTIVE MASSAGE

4 · INTRODUCTION

When I massage Mary Decker's surgically scarred legs, the massage always produces a pained smile. The slight pain comes from the pressure I am putting on Mary's powerful muscles. The smile comes from the knowledge that this sometimes blessed agony is actually good for her. She knows that with each push of my thumbs, the chemical wastes and excess fluids caused by hard training are being squeezed out of her muscles.

Although the massage sometimes hurts, Mary knows that it revitalizes her tired muscles with fresh blood and fluids, making them feel as new as a two-day layoff would. As she has said many times, "Without massage, I wouldn't be running nearly as well as I am. It has reduced the number of injuries and their severity when they happen."

Reducing the number and severity of injuries is exactly what massage is supposed to do, which is why it is "preventive." Without it, injuries would be more frequent and long-lasting; hard workouts would yield to stiff muscles; soreness would be a way of life.

Most athletes—even "weekend warriors"—suffer from soreness. You will be glad to know that the massage techniques in the following chapters will help ease that soreness immediately by speeding the movement of fluid through the muscles, thereby reducing swelling; removing the harmful chemicals of exertion from the muscles, thereby reducing pain; and making the muscles more pliable, thereby preparing the athlete for a quicker return to activity.

Preventive massage may be administered as often as desired, with no fear of "overdose." And, since it requires no special knowledge of anatomy, it can be effectively administered by almost anyone who studies the proper techniques. However, so you don't spend all of your spare time giving or receiving massages, I have included massage schedules later in this chapter, organized by various sports and the muscles affected by them. These will help you know when and where to massage. But remember that the way the muscles feel is the best guide.

Anyone with any of the following symptoms can probably benefit from the "painful pleasure" of preventive athletic massage:

• *Recurring injury:* Is there an Achilles tendon that always hurts after a run? How about tennis elbow? Massage may loosen up some severely tightened muscles that are creating tendon irritation.

• *Chronic stiffness:* Do certain muscles feel as though they are bound by bandages? Preventive massage may remove some of the muscle tension or edema build-up that causes this feeling of tightness.

• *Sore spots:* Perhaps lactic acid build-up has caused muscle tension that won't go away. Preventive massage can take the pressure off tears in the muscle fibers and get rid of that lactic acid marinade, both of which cause soreness.

• *Chronic pain:* Preventive massage can soften the scar tissue that irritates surrounding tissue to cause painful muscle spasms.

Follow these guidelines to be certain that the massage you give is safe and effective:

• *Use deep strokes on muscle only.* Do not apply deep strokes to the connective tissue, which is the narrow area near the ends of the muscles, such as the Achilles tendon or the point where the biceps inserts into the elbow. To do so may damage tendons and ligaments. To play it safe, restrict your deep strokes to the bulky portion of the muscle to avoid causing or worsening an injury. There are other strokes that can safely be used on connective tissues.

• *Do not exceed the point of pain.* Although deep strokes and cross-fiber strokes will be painful at first, even when administered with light pressure, don't apply more pressure than is comfortable for the athlete. Not only do you run the risk of injuring the area, but the athlete will tense those muscles, which will reduce the effectiveness of the massage.

• *Glide from one stroke to another.* Make the massage a smooth experience by maintaining skin contact with the athlete.

• *Don't forget the oil.* Comfort and effectiveness depend upon proper lubrication.

• *Follow the instructions for each body part as given.* The order of the strokes has not been chosen at random. Each stroke prepares the muscle for the next movement, one building upon the other to cause increased

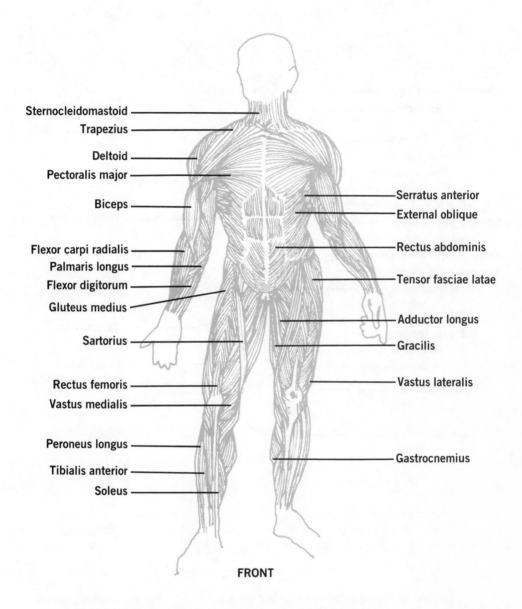

Sternocleidomastoid
Trapezius
Deltoid
Pectoralis major
Biceps
Flexor carpi radialis
Palmaris longus
Flexor digitorum
Gluteus medius
Sartorius
Rectus femoris
Vastus medialis
Peroneus longus
Tibialis anterior
Soleus

Serratus anterior
External oblique
Rectus abdominis
Tensor fasciae latae
Adductor longus
Gracilis
Vastus lateralis
Gastrocnemius

FRONT

blood flow, or hyperemia. As your technique improves, you may want to vary the routine according to the needs and wants of the athlete. In the beginning, however, the best results can be derived by following the instructions exactly.

• *Finally, some problems take time to heal.* Muscular tension, especially the type that involves knots caused by scar tissue, cannot be worked out quickly or simply. Patience is required. Slow, firm pressure, rather than impatient probing, will make muscle tension yield more quickly.

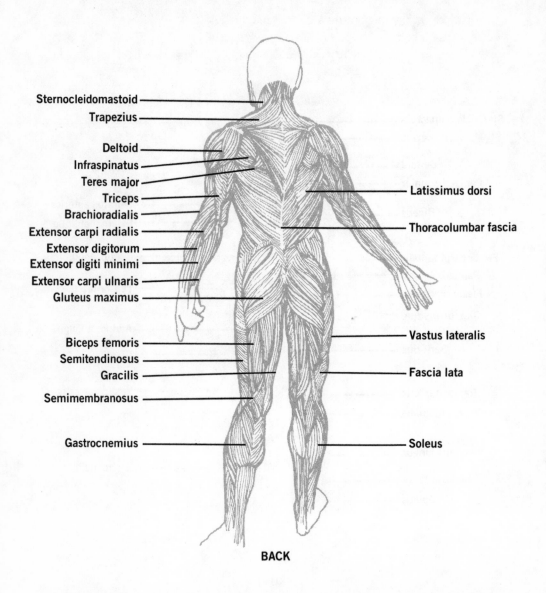

Sternocleidomastoid

Trapezius

Deltoid

Infraspinatus

Teres major

Triceps

Brachioradialis

Extensor carpi radialis

Extensor digitorum

Extensor digiti minimi

Extensor carpi ulnaris

Gluteus maximus

Biceps femoris

Semitendinosus

Gracilis

Semimembranosus

Gastrocnemius

Latissimus dorsi

Thoracolumbar fascia

Vastus lateralis

Fascia lata

Soleus

BACK

Full body massage takes forty-five minutes to an hour to do properly, but you don't have to do the full body every time you do a massage. Runners, for instance, get most of their stress in the legs and back, since running uses those muscles almost exclusively. And swimmers require massage of the shoulders and neck for all the pulling and twisting of those regions. So, for runners, most massages can just cover the legs and back, while swimmers need their necks and shoulders massaged more than other areas.

Since I massage a large number of athletes each day, I offer them the choice of an upper- or lower-body massage. They make the choice on the basis of which area is in greatest need of attention.

To help you work on the area that needs the massage, I have divided the demonstration chapters for preventive massage into body parts: hands and arms, chest, abdomen, legs (front and back), feet, buttocks, back and neck. You can turn to the section dealing with the appropriate body part and follow the illustrations and directions.

Different sports will require different massage regimens. If an area is sore, it should be massaged. If there is no noticeable soreness, then follow these guidelines, according to the sport involved:

Running

Because running is the act of pushing the body forward, the muscles that are used the most are those in the back of the legs, particularly the calves. The front of the legs and the lower back are also used a lot. Although they receive none of the pounding that the legs and back do, the shoulders may also need occasional massage to relieve the effects of arm-swinging, and the neck may also become tense, depending upon an individual's running style.

Massage schedule: For the person who runs at least five times per week, I recommend full massage of the legs three times per week. Also, the feet, back and shoulders need massage at least once a week.

For the person who runs less than five times per week, two full leg massages should suffice, but the back and shoulders should be massaged once a week.

Swimming

Swimming is primarily the act of pulling oneself through the water. The muscles that do that pulling are in the arms and shoulders. Those muscles should receive attention first, followed by those in the neck, which sometimes undergo considerable strain from twisting. Another area that requires occasional attention on a swimmer is the abdomen, which is sometimes strained by the constant reaching action. Surprisingly, the legs rarely need massage, since the water they kick provides a sort of massaging action itself.

Massage schedule: For the frequent swimmer (at least four times per week), the arms, shoulders and chest should be massaged at least twice per week, with one of those sessions including massage of the neck and abdomen. One massage per week should be done on the legs, with special attention being paid to the lower legs and Achilles tendons.

Bicycling

The muscles most obviously affected by this sport are in the legs, primarily the thighs, which provide most of the pushing action. Next are the muscles of the back, especially the lower back, which strain from the bent-over position of the cyclist. The neck and shoulders become fatigued—particularly the neck, which tires from the rider's need to look up.

Massage schedule: Massage should be performed on the front and back of the legs and on the lower back after each hard cycling workout. At least one massage per week, but more if necessary, should be devoted to the upper back, shoulders, arms and neck.

Court Sports

Racquetball, handball and squash affect a large number of muscles, including those of the shoulders, back, arms and legs. All that twisting sometimes affects the abdomen, too. And if the athlete is one of those players who push off with their feet, don't forget them in the massage routine.

Massage schedule: Leg massage should be performed after games, with special attention being paid to the feet. The entire upper body and the abdomen should be massaged at least once a week.

Weight Lifting

Most "weight people" work the upper body one day and the lower body the next, to avoid overuse of an area. Still these muscles tire and require massage.

Massage schedule: Massage the muscles on the days they are exercised. For instance, when the athlete lifts weights with the upper body, massage the arms, chest, shoulders, upper back and neck. On the days he works the lower body, massage the legs, lower back and abdomen.

Skiing

Of course, the legs of a skier need massage, as do the back and arms, which are probably used more by cross-country than downhill skiers.

Massage schedule: Most skiers are weekend athletes and will require full body massage to recover from a day of unusually hard activity. For the frequent skier—one who skis at least three times per week—the legs and lower back should be massaged twice a week. In addition, the arms, shoulders and upper back should be done once a week.

Backpacking

Depending upon the load carried in the pack, you will want to pay special attention to the back and the abdomen, which experience considerable strain from carrying packs. And don't forget the legs and feet. A massage in the midst of a beautiful outdoor setting is a sweet delight, so don't forget to pack the book.

Massage schedule: Massage of the legs and lower back is a must after almost all backpack ventures. And, if the pack is a heavy one, don't forget to massage the shoulders, chest, neck and even the abdomen.

Baseball/Softball

As the main sport of "the weekend warrior," baseball was responsible for many of my patients' complaints when I was in private practice. Mainly, the complaints were about stretched muscles and sore shoulders from throwing the ball and swinging the bat, but anyone who managed to get a hit complained about sore legs from running the bases.

Massage schedule: Baseball should be followed by full massage of the legs and, if needed, massage of the lower back, arms and shoulders.

Basketball

What's true for baseball players is true for basketball players, only to a greater degree. Depending upon how aggressively it is played, basketball works all the body's muscles, especially the legs, which undergo the stresses of start-and-stop play, and the arms and shoulders, which receive wear and tear every time the player goes for a basket.

Massage schedule: Basketball games should be followed by full leg massage as well as massage of the feet and lower back. Massage of the upper back, shoulders, neck and arms are optional, depending on need.

Field Sports

Sports like soccer, football and rugby usually take a toll on the body that only a full body massage can remedy. It is usually easy to spot the areas that need the greatest attention. They are the ones that are the sorest.

Massage schedule: Field sports almost always require full leg massage after a game, as well as massage of the lower back and buttocks. Other areas that may require attention are the neck and shoulders, depending on the degree of soreness the athlete is experiencing.

Bowling

Due to the weight of the ball, the arm receives much of the straining and stretching in bowling. The lower back also receives stress, because of the bending necessary to roll the ball.

Massage schedule: Follow bowling with full massage of the legs, lower back and arms, especially the one used to throw the ball. Also perform shoulder and neck massage if the bowler feels they are needed.

Some of you may now be ready to move on to the actual massage procedures. Others may need a quick review of the strokes referred to in the previous chapter. I'll cover the important strokes again briefly. If you need further explanation, reread the preceding chapter.

Three movements accomplish about 95 percent of the desired effect:

• *Deep stroking:* The thumbs run parallel to the grain of the muscle, spreading the fibers through compression.

• *Cross-fiber stroking:* Working across the grain with the thumbs at a 90-degree angle to the body, spread each fiber away from its neighbor. This is the only way of stretching a muscle across its breadth, and is also the most effective way of breaking adhesions that stick muscles together.

• *Jostling:* Loosely grab a muscle group between the thumb and fingers, softly squeezing and shaking it from the point of origin (closest to the heart) to insertion (farthest from the heart). This is the movement for relaxation.

Finally, a few words about musculature. In the photographs which follow, I have used runners Mary Decker, Alberto Salazar and Margaret Groos as models. Because they run an extraordinary number of miles each day, they have a very low percentage of body fat. As a result, their muscles stand out in sharp relief and are very easy to find.

Your body, or the body of the person you are working on, may be different due to a higher percentage of body fat. So you may not be able to see the muscles on someone else as easily as you see the ones in this book. If that is the case, rely on your sense of touch. By probing the skin, you should easily be able to feel the outline of the muscles. Everyone's muscles are in the same places, so use these pictures as a road map of the body.

One more thing: the instructions *upper hand* and *lower hand* refer to where your hands are in relation to the athlete's body: *upper hand* means the hand in the direction of the athlete's head and *lower hand* means the hand in the direction of the athlete's feet.

5 · HANDS AND ARMS

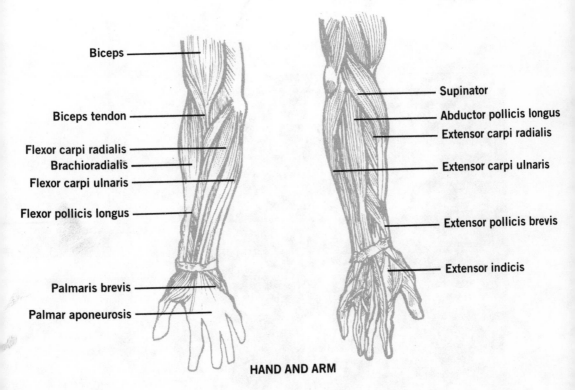

Biceps

Biceps tendon

Flexor carpi radialis

Brachioradialis

Flexor carpi ulnaris

Flexor pollicis longus

Palmaris brevis

Palmar aponeurosis

Supinator

Abductor pollicis longus

Extensor carpi radialis

Extensor carpi ulnaris

Extensor pollicis brevis

Extensor indicis

HAND AND ARM

The hand is an incredibly versatile mechanism made up of a complex mass of tendons and tiny muscles. Movement of the thumb, for instance, is controlled by eight separate muscles and tendons. The skin that covers it is specialized, with a thick, tough, firmly attached palm on one side for gripping and loose-fitting skin on the other to allow the muscles and tendons free movement.

Since the hand is largely controlled by the more than fifteen tendons that extend from the forearm, it makes sense to massage the hand and arm as one unit. These tendons, some of them enclosed in sheaths, allow the hand to grip. When they tire, so does the hand they control.

Rarely do the muscles of the hand and fingers suffer from fatigue injuries in athletics. Also, since the muscles of the hand and fingers are small and intricate, there are a limited number of strokes which can be applied to them. But even at that, hand massage is a delight.

The arm, too, is a pleasure to have massaged, with one major difference from the hand—it isn't as delicate. And that allows you to use the deeper strokes.

The arm consists of upper arm muscles, called the biceps and triceps, which narrow where their tendons attach at the elbow. The biceps flexes the arm and the triceps straightens it out.

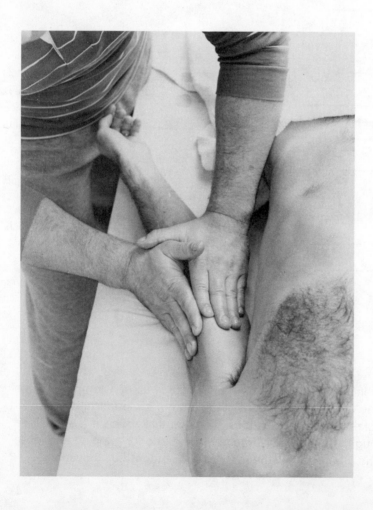

The forearm has two main sets of muscles, too. The flexor pronator group draws the hand toward the wrist and the extensor supinator group straightens it out.

These groups of muscles join on the outside and inside of the elbow. Irritation of these muscles causes the conditions known as "tennis elbow" and "pitcher's elbow." These two problems may be avoided by preventive massage. If you already have them, refer to the chapter on curative massage of the arm and hand (Chapter 17, "Tennis Elbow").

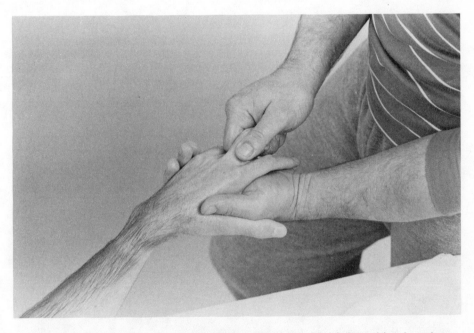

Broad Cross-Fiber Stroking of the Fingers Hold the athlete's palm in yours, with the fingers draped over the side of your hand. Pick up each finger, rubbing it between your thumb and fingers on the length of the finger. Repeat three times on all the fingers and thumb.

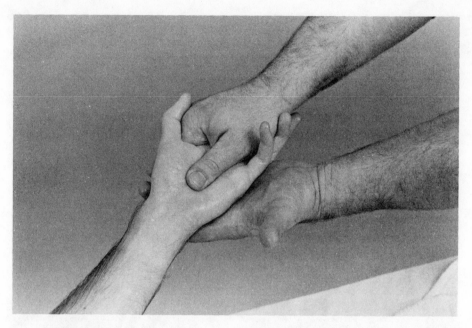

Broad Cross-Fiber Stroking of the Palm   With the athlete's hand palm up in yours, use your thumb to cross the palm from one side to the other. Repeat this motion at least three times, covering the entire palm each time.

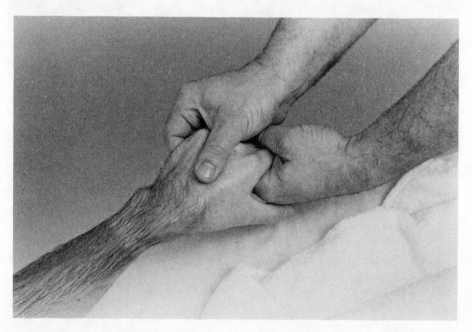

Broad Cross-Fiber Stroking of the Back of the Hand   Place the athlete's hand palm down in yours, holding the fingers with your thumb and fingers. Using the thumb of your other hand, stroke across the back of the hand in rows moving from the wrist to the knuckles. Repeat this movement at least three times.

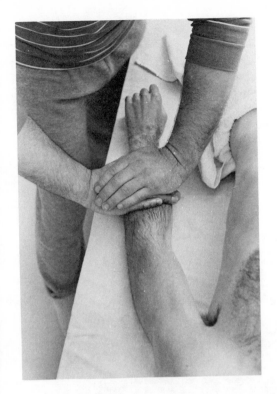

Light Stroking of the Arm With the athlete's arm flat on the table, place the palms of your hands on top of each other (for more controlled pressure) and stroke gently up the arm to the top of the shoulder. Slide your palms back down the arm and repeat the procedure, this time more firmly. A third time—still more firmly—should cause that rush of blood known as hyperemia. Turn the palm up and repeat the procedure.

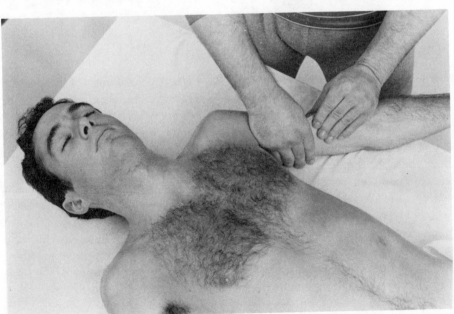

Kneading of the Arm From a position next to the athlete's shoulder, using the thumbs and fingers of both hands, knead the arm from the wrist to the biceps, and then back down again. After the arm has been kneaded up and down three times, repeat the light stroking twice to ready the arm for the next movement.

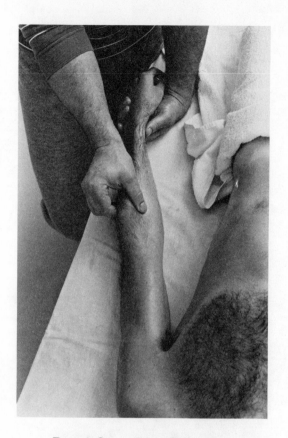

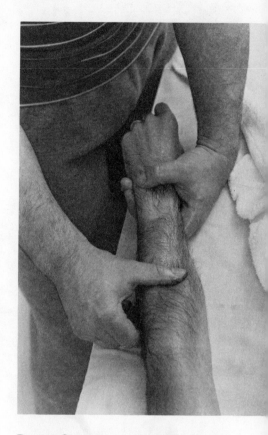

Broad Cross-Fiber Stroking of the Forearm From a position next to the athlete's hip, hold the athlete's hand palm down with your lower hand to keep the arm stationary. Use your thumb to stroke across the muscles of the athlete's forearm, from the wrist to the elbow. Since the thumb will only cover about an inch with each stroke, several strokes will be required to go from the wrist to the elbow. Repeat this three times. Then turn the palm up and repeat the broad cross-fiber strokes across the inside of the forearm.

Deep Stroking of the Forearm Holding the hand palm down, stroke deeply with the thumb in a straight line from the wrist to the elbow. Work around the forearm in approximately one-inch strips. Don't stroke too deeply on the first pass, but administer more pressure with each pass over the area. Cover the top of the forearm three times. Then turn the athlete's hand palm up and repeat the deep stroking on the inside of the forearm.

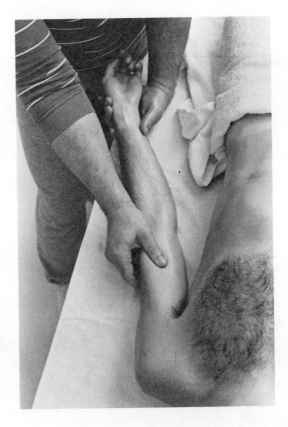

Broad Cross-Fiber Stroking of the Upper Arm Still standing next to the athlete's hip, hold the athlete's wrist with the hand palm up. Stroke across the biceps with the thumb. You are moving across the muscle, so it will require several passes to move up the arm from the elbow to the top of the biceps. Cover the upper arm, including the shoulder (deltoid). Repeat this procedure at least three times, remembering to increase thumb pressure with each pass.

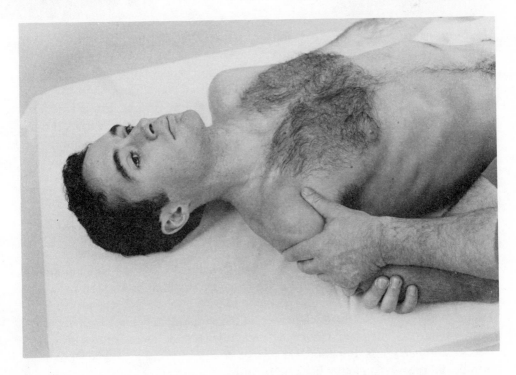

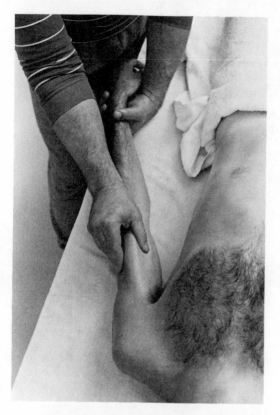
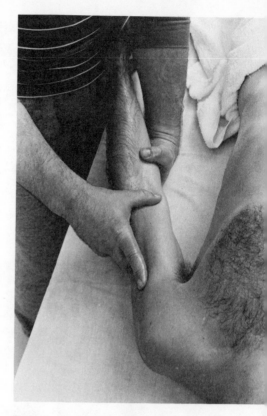

Jostling of the Biceps Hold the athlete's wrist for stability and grasp the biceps with the thumb and fingers, shaking, or "jostling," it gently, until it feels loose and relaxed. Repeat this three times, with each jostle lasting at least five seconds.

Deep Stroking of the Upper Arm Firmly grasping the athlete's forearm with your lower hand, use the thumb of your upper hand to stroke up the arm deeply. Repeat at least three times, covering in rows the inside and outside of the upper arm. Do not exceed the point of pain but do try deeper strokes with each session.

Deep Stroking of the Shoulder (See facing page, above.) Holding the cap of the shoulder (deltoid) with both hands, use the thumbs to deep-stroke the front and side of the shoulder, stroking toward the head. Cover as much area as possible, leaving the back portion of the shoulder until the athlete turns over for the back massage. Cover the area at least three times, progressively deeper with each pass. Repeat these strokes on the front of the athlete's other arm before proceeding to the back of the arm.

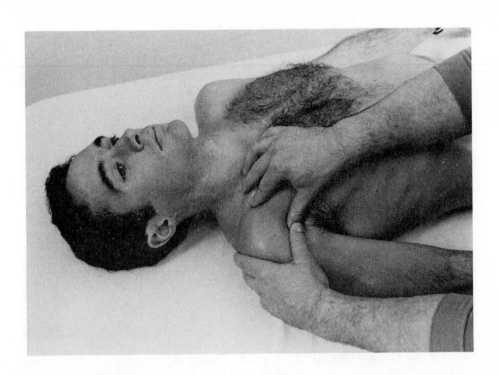

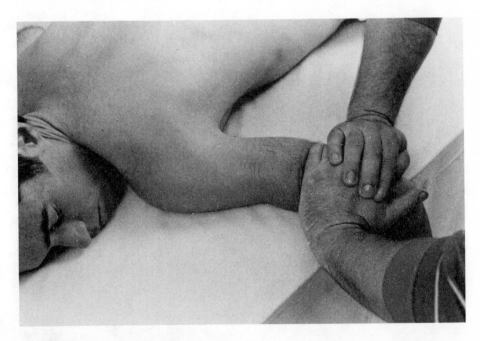

Light Stroking of the Triceps With the athlete's arm to the side or dangling from the table, put one palm over the other on the triceps and stroke toward the shoulder. Repeat three times, gliding back to the elbow after each stroke.

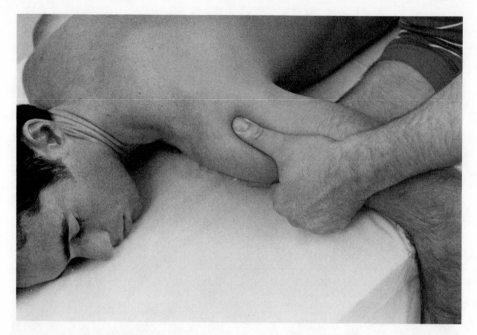

Broad Cross-Fiber Stroking of the Upper Arm   With one hand held under the arm for stability, stroke around the arm in rows with the thumb of the other hand, from the elbow to the top of the deltoid muscle. Repeat three times.

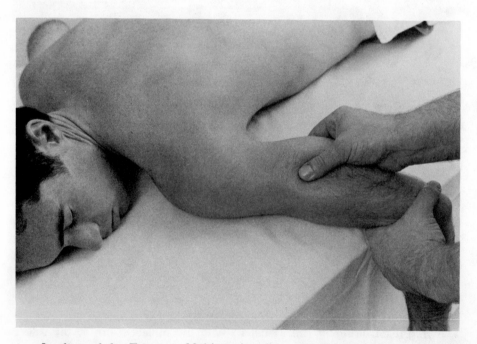

Jostling of the Triceps   Holding the elbow for stability with your upper hand, grasp the athlete's triceps between the thumb and fingers of the other hand and jostle it vigorously for about five seconds. Repeat three times.

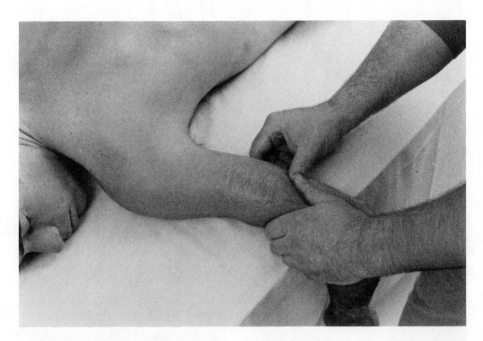

Deep Stroking of the Triceps Holding the upper arm between your fingers for stability, place your thumbs on top of each other and stroke the back of the arm in rows from the elbow to the shoulder. Cover the entire back of the arm with strokes. Repeat three times.

Conclude the massage with light stroking of the entire arm from wrist to shoulder, and repeat the massage on the back of the other arm.

6 · CHEST

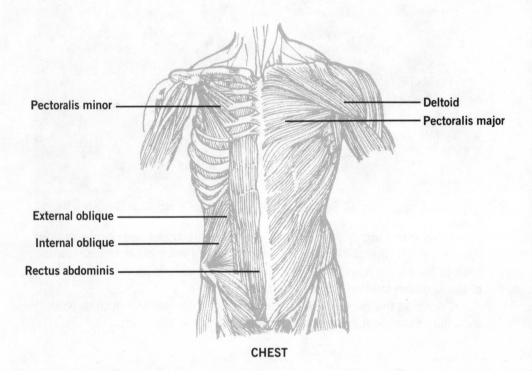

Pectoralis minor

Deltoid

Pectoralis major

External oblique

Internal oblique

Rectus abdominis

CHEST

The chest is a latticework of muscles, covered on each side by the thick, broad, triangular muscles known as the pectoralis majors. Beneath those muscles are the pectoralis minors, thin, flat triangles of muscle that attach to the ribs near the collarbone (clavicle.) Another muscle, the subclavius, is between the collarbone and the first rib.

These muscles move the arms up and down and across the chest, and they make possible pushing movements and shoulder movements.

Because of all that these muscles do, and the many tendon attachments they have to the ribs and shoulders, they should be kept loose, especially for body builders and weight lifters, who subject this area to an extraordinary amount of stress.

Light Stroking of the Chest
Standing next to the athlete's hip, place the palms at the base of the rib cage and stroke lightly up the center of the chest (sternum) to the base of the collarbone and then back. Perform the same movement again, beginning at the outer edges of the chest and covering the outside of the rib cage, to the base of the ribs and then back. On women, these strokes should move between and around the breasts, as should all movements in this area on women. Cover the chest three times with these light strokes before progressing to the next movement.

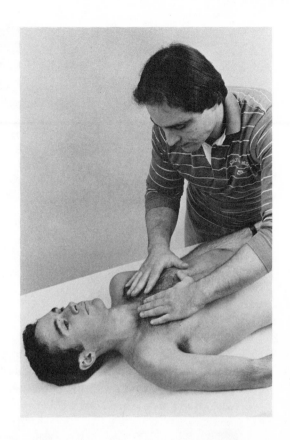

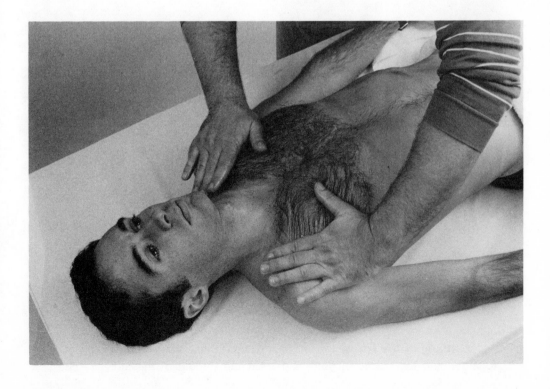

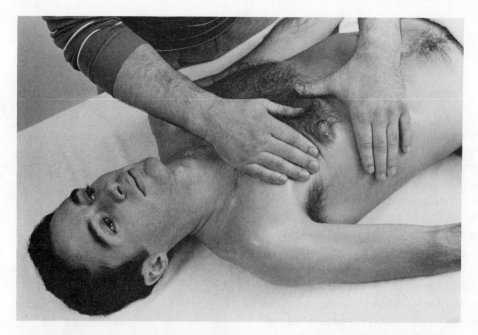

Kneading of the Chest Standing next to the chest, reach across the athlete and begin kneading the far side of the chest from the collarbone to the ribs, making sure to cover the entire half of the chest. Knead the entire half at least three times. Then switch sides and knead the other half of the chest.

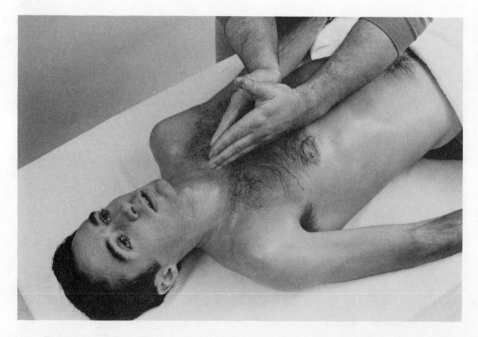

Fanning of the Chest From next to the athlete's hip, place your palms together and the edges of your hands on the middle of the athlete's chest

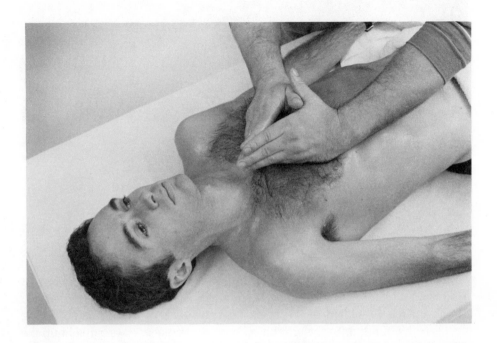

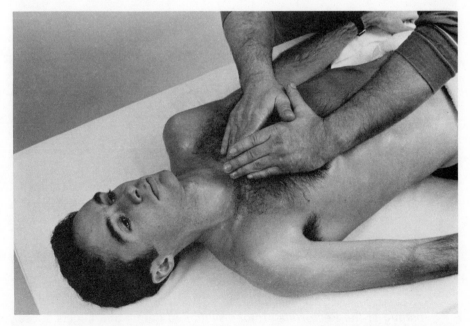

(sternum). Applying pressure, fan the hands out toward the edge of the athlete's chest and glide back again. Repeat until the entire chest is covered, moving up a hand-length at a time. Perform the procedure three times before going on to the next movement.

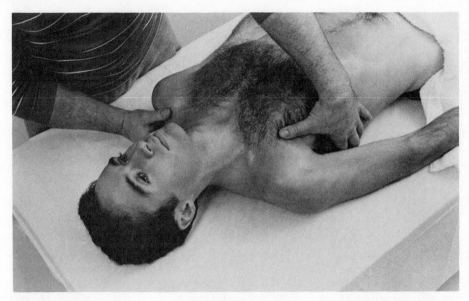

Broad Cross-Fiber Stroking of the Major Chest Muscles (Pectoralis Major) Standing next to the chest, reach across the athlete and place your thumb on the centerline of the chest near the base of the rib cage. Stroke deeply with your thumbs toward the collarbone. Stroke in rows, straight up the chest, moving a thumb-width at a time toward the armpit. Cover the pectoralis muscles three times with this stroke. Repeat on the other side of the chest.

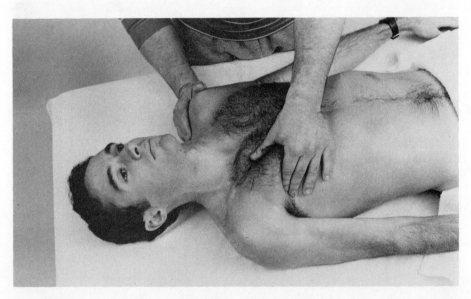

Jostling of the Pectoralis Major With your thumb and fingers, loosely hold the pectoralis muscle at the junction of the armpit and shoulder. Shake the muscle for at least five seconds. Repeat this movement three times on one side of the chest before performing it on the other. Both sides may be jostled simultaneously if you wish.

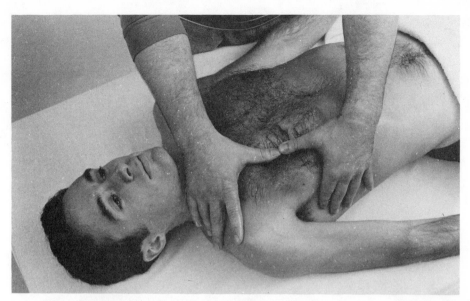

Deep Stroking of the Pectoralis Major   From a position next to the chest, reach across the athlete and place your fingers tip to tip on the center of the chest, near the collarbone. Stroke out to the armpit and glide the thumbs back. Repeat the stroke about an inch farther down the chest. Continue until the pectoralis has been covered to the base of the rib cage. Then work your way in rows back to the collarbone. Repeat three times; then do the other side.

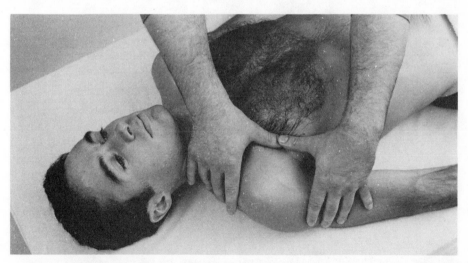

Deep Stroking of the Pectoralis Minor   Standing next to the athlete's shoulder, place one thumb on top of the other, about an inch to the inside of the athlete's shoulder. Pull the thumbs toward the base of the rib cage in a direct line. One stroke to an area about two inches above the base of the ribs will cover this muscle, since it is narrow. Repeat three times and then do the other side of the chest.

   Finish by covering the entire chest with light strokes by the palms of the hands to enhance blood circulation.

7 · ABDOMEN

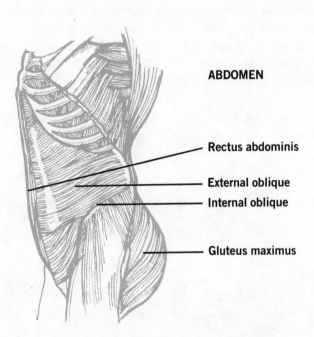

ABDOMEN

Rectus abdominis

External oblique

Internal oblique

Gluteus maximus

In massage of the abdomen, we are primarily concerned with the superficial muscles, those closest to the skin that cover the deep muscles protecting the organs. They are the muscles involved extensively in athletic activity and can be safely massaged.

The deep muscles of the abdomen benefit from massage of the superficial muscles. Direct deep massage of the abdomen is best conducted by a professional, since it involves working through a layer of muscle.

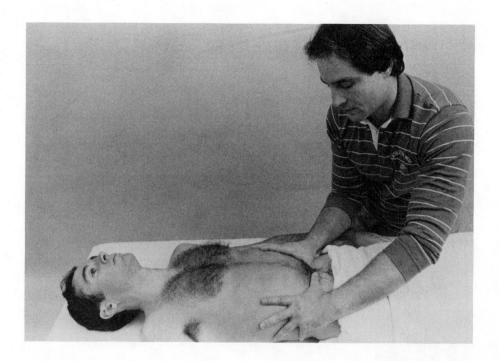

We are interested in massaging the stretching and straining muscles of this area, particularly those muscles known as the obliques. They are the largest of the abdomen's three flat muscles and cover the ribs at what most of us consider "the tickle zone."

Although the muscles of this area remain limber (probably from the movements of breathing), they are sometimes subject to pulls from making the big reach in sports like baseball, or traumatic contact injury from sports like soccer.

Because it *is* the tickle zone for some, the muscles of the ribs are often impossible to massage.

Another possible tickle zone on an athlete is the rectus abdominis, the long and flat (if we are lucky) muscle that extends the entire length of the abdomen, from the pubic area to the base of the rib cage. It is attached by tendons to the ribs, which may at times suffer some strain.

The abdominals are usually an athlete's weakest muscles. Because of that, work the area lightly at first, making sure not to apply more pressure than is comfortable.

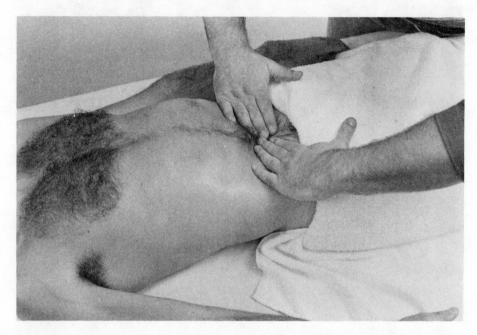

Light Stroking of the Abdomen From a position next to the athlete's hip, stroke the athlete's abdomen with your palms, from just below the navel to the base of the rib cage. Repeat this several times, making sure to cover the entire abdomen. Instead of this movement, you can substitute petrissage, the light, circular movements of the fingertips. The purpose of this first movement is to prepare for the deeper movements and to desensitize the area so it won't be so ticklish.

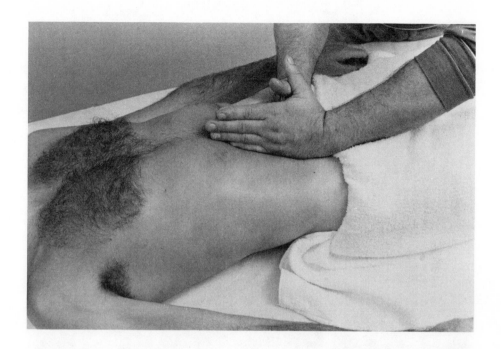

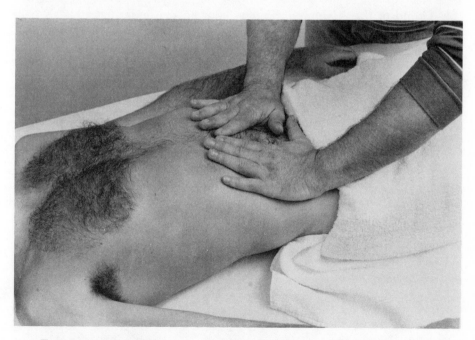

Fanning of the Abdomen   Placing your hands together at the midline of the abdomen, fan out its edges, applying pressure as you stroke out to the athlete's sides. Glide the hands back together and repeat the stroke. Be sure to cover the entire abdomen, from the base of the chest to just below the navel. Repeat at least three times.

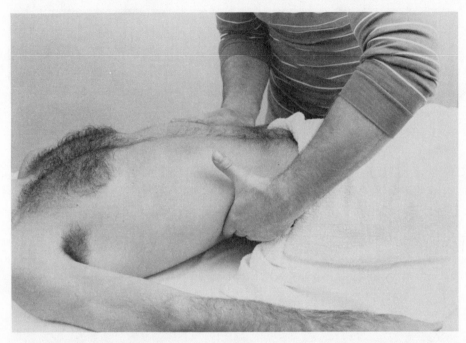

Lifting of the Abdomen Putting your fingers under the athlete's back and as close to the spine as possible, lift and pull the tissue as you withdraw your hands. Repeat this three times over the small of the back, from the base of the ribs to the pelvis.

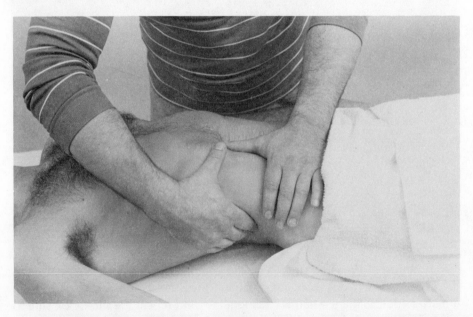

Kneading of the Abdomen From a position next to the athlete's abdomen, reach across and grasp the athlete's side, just above the hip. Squeeze your hands together alternately, kneading from the hipbone over the ribs to the base of the armpit and back down again. Repeat three times and then knead the abdomen itself, from the base of the rib cage to just below the navel and back again. Repeat that movement three times. Move to the other side of the athlete and repeat these kneading movements.

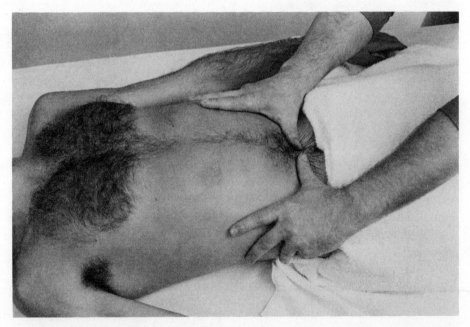

Deep Stroking of the Abdomen   From beside the athlete's hip, place your hands on either side of the abdomen, fingers draped over the outer edges and thumbs across the inner abdomen. Begin stroking with the thumbs just beneath the navel and continue to the rib cage. Cover the entire abdomen lengthwise.

Caution: The abdomen is a complex maze of muscles that cover many delicate organs. Be sure not to apply more pressure than the athlete is comfortable with.

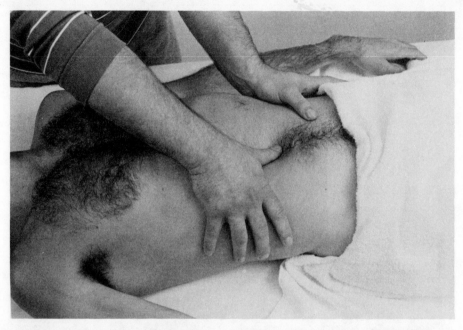

Broad Cross-Fiber Stroking of the Abdomen   From a position next to the athlete's shoulder, reach across the abdomen with the upper hand, placing your thumb on the abdomen's midline and your fingers over the outer abdomen. Then stroke from the midline to the outer edge of the abdomen with the pad of your thumb. Several of those strokes will be required to cover the abdomen from below the navel to the rib cage. Cover the area at least three times, then perform the same movements on the other side.

When both sides are completed, cover the entire abdomen with light stroking of the palms.

8 · LEGS (Front and Back)

The muscles of the leg run the gamut from the largest in the body to the smallest, the strongest to the weakest. The leg contains the power of mobility, which enables us to do almost everything we do athletically. It also contains the knee, a joint so vulnerable that many describe it as "God's mistake" in making the human body.

At the top of the leg is the thigh, with the quadriceps, the largest muscle in the body. The thigh also contains the body's longest muscle, the hamstring. There are several lesser muscles between them, each subject to just as great a likelihood of injury as the larger muscles.

The quadriceps are important to explosive movement, like that seen in sprinting, racquetball and soccer, while the hamstring muscles are especially important to long-distance runners.

Because of the size and toughness of most athletes' thighs, you will have to use more pressure during preventive massage. And because of the importance of these muscles to athletes, it is best to massage the legs first in a full body massage—particularly the thighs—while your hands are strong.

The knee is a delicate combination of ligaments that hold the large leg-bones together, a cartilage that cushions the bones, and a kneecap, or patella, which is the protective plate of bone in front of the joint. It is both a hinge and lever, capable of great flexibility at times and inflexibility at others.

The muscles from the thigh and lower leg all join at the knee.

Preventive massage of the thigh can keep the tendons and ligaments loose and can increase joint flexibility. Reduced tension in the joint greatly diminishes the likelihood of a number of hip and knee disorders common in sports. These

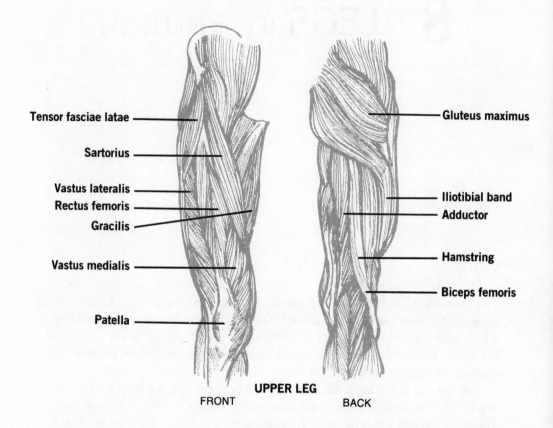

Tensor fasciae latae

Sartorius

Vastus lateralis

Rectus femoris

Gracilis

Vastus medialis

Patella

Gluteus maximus

Iliotibial band

Adductor

Hamstring

Biceps femoris

UPPER LEG
FRONT   BACK

include patella tendinitis, strains in the hip, injuries of the iliotibial band (outer thigh) and runner's knee.

At the bottom of the leg are the calf muscle (in back) and the shin (in front). Because so many sports make extraordinary demands on this part of the leg, preventive massage can play an important role in its maintenance.

Remember, this is the part of the body that contains the Achilles tendon, the body's largest—and some feel most important—tendon. Any tendon is weakest at the point at which it attaches to the muscle. Because it is worked every time we walk or run, it is this tendon and the adjoining muscles that do the most work of any of the body's voluntary muscles.

The hamstring, too, is subject to injury in most sports, mostly due to the

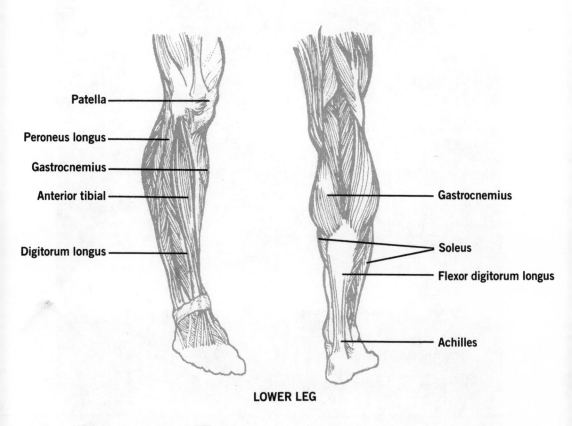

Patella

Peroneus longus

Gastrocnemius

Anterior tibial

Digitorum longus

Gastrocnemius

Soleus

Flexor digitorum longus

Achilles

LOWER LEG

fact that it is not used to its fullest until called upon to perform at optimal capacity in athletic competiton. When this happens, the hamstring is subject to strain.

Once fatigue of the muscle has set in, the hamstring loses its ability to relax following a constriction. The opposing muscle (quadriceps) being stronger, the contracted hamstring will be forced to extend farther, causing or worsening a hamstring pull.

Preventive massage lengthens the muscles and prevents the shortening that leads to pulling away from attachments or tearing fibers. It will also keep blood moving through an area that experiences many torn fibers in the course of strenuous training.

Front of the Leg

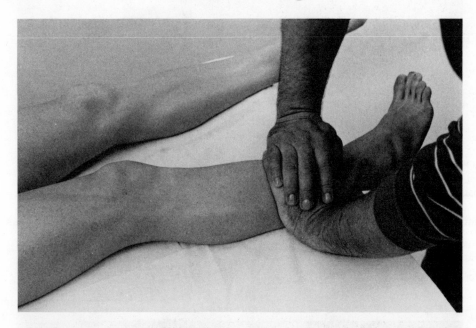

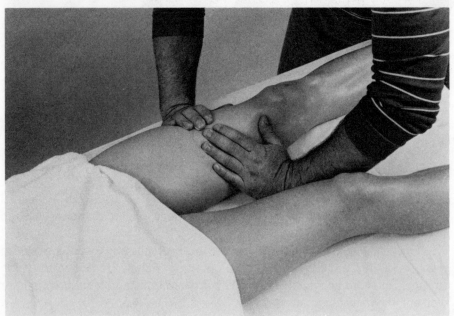

Light Stroking of the Leg From a position by the foot, stroke the entire leg in one movement with the hands flat, from the ankle to the thigh. Pressure should be firm during this stroke, but not deep. Glide your hands back down the leg and repeat the movement. This stroke should be done four times or until the athlete's skin becomes warm.

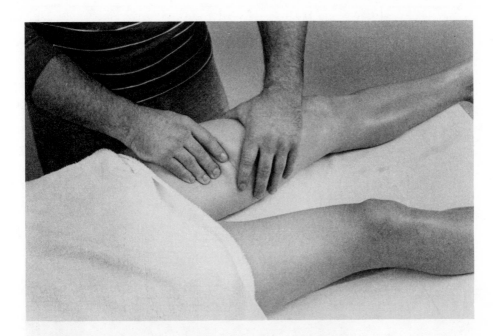

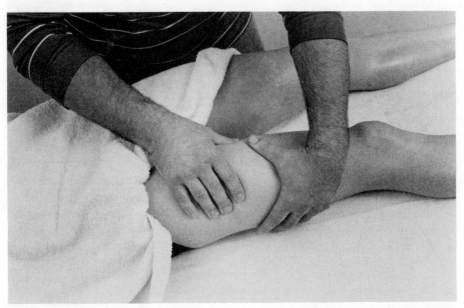

Kneading of the Leg From a position next to the athlete's legs, knead the inside of the near leg from the ankle to the crotch and back again. Make sure to cover the inside of the leg and the top of the thigh as well. These are large muscles and should be worked with considerable force. Don't be afraid to lift them from the bone so even deeper muscles can be milked of waste products. Repeat this movement three times and then knead the outside of the far leg, kneading from the ankle to the crotch and back again.

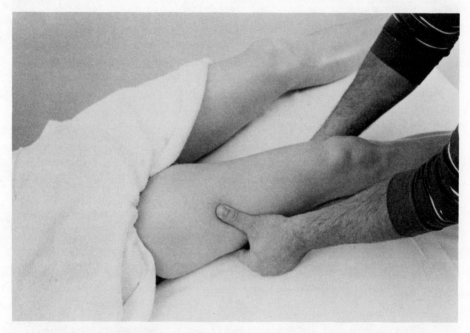

Broad Cross-Fiber Stroking of the Outermost Section of the Upper Leg (Iliotibial Band) Standing next to the athlete's knee, stabilize the leg closest to you with the lower hand. In your mind, divide the front of the leg into four equal quadrants. (Dividing the leg into sections makes it easier to work those massive muscles.) With the thumb of your upper hand, begin administering the broad cross-fiber strokes to the outermost section of the top of the leg, which begins at the hip and runs in a strip to the knee. Cover this section up and down at least three times.

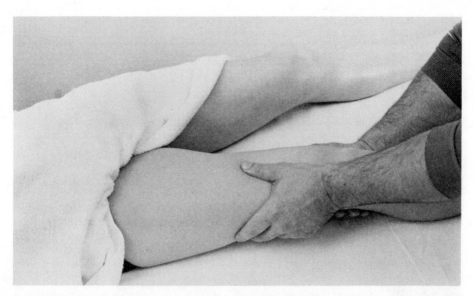

Broad Cross-Fiber Stroking of the Second Section (Rectus Femoris and Vastus Lateralis) This area is shown in the illustration on page 68. Still stabilizing the closest leg with the lower hand on the inside of the knee, stroke across this section with the thumb of the upper hand, moving in rows from the hip to just above the kneecap, covering this section up and down at least three times.

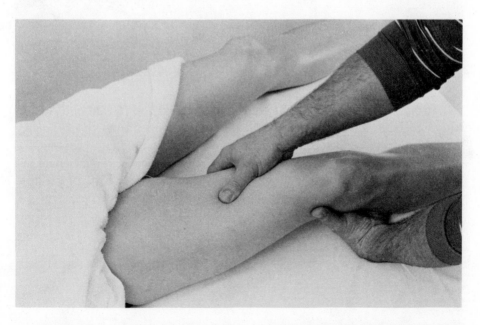

Broad Cross-Fiber Stroking of the Third Section (Rectus Femoris and Vastus Medialis) Stabilize the athlete's leg with the upper hand on the outside of the knee. With the lower hand, stroke across the third section with the thumb, from the hip to just above the knee. Work this area up and down at least three times.

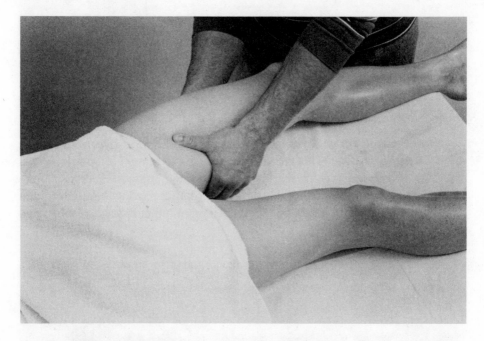

Broad Cross-Fiber Stroking of the Fourth Section (Groin and Adductors) Stabilize the athlete's leg with the upper hand on the outside of the thigh. Stroke across the section nearest the crotch with the thumb crossing the muscle fibers in rows, from the crotch to the knee and back again. Repeat this movement at least three times. Upon completion of the massage of the front of the upper leg, jostle the thigh vigorously to relax it for the next movement.

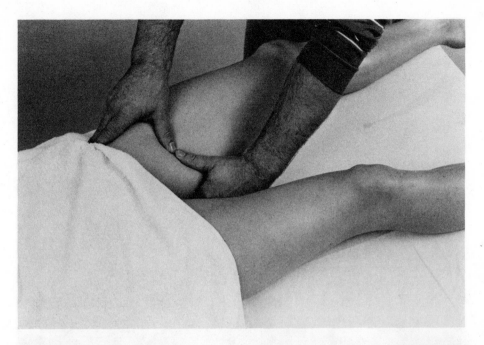

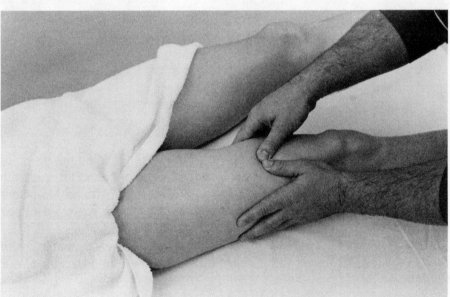

Deep Stroking of the Front of the Upper Leg From next to the athlete's knee, put your fingers on either side of the athlete's thigh and bring the tips of the thumbs together. Deep-stroke the second through the fourth sections. Cover the same areas you covered with the broad cross-fiber movements, excluding the iliotibial band (section one) and the patella tendon, that area directly above the kneecap. These are areas of delicate connective tissue. To prevent them from tearing, they should not be deep-stroked. Cover the other sections at least three times each.

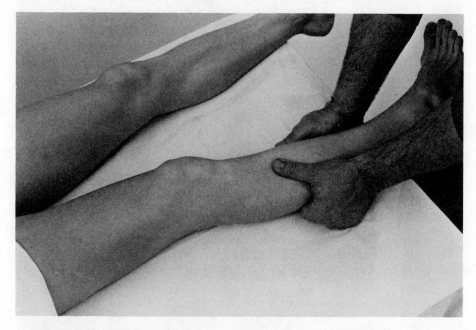

Broad Cross-Fiber Stroking of the Lower Leg   Holding the inside of the calf with the inside hand, use the thumb of the other hand to stroke the outermost edge of the shin muscle to the shinbone with broad cross-fiber strokes. Cross the entire area in rows, from the ankle to the base of the knee and back again until the area has been covered three times.

Muscles on the inside of the lower leg are most effectively treated from the back of the leg. Treatment with these strokes from the front may bring about shin splints.

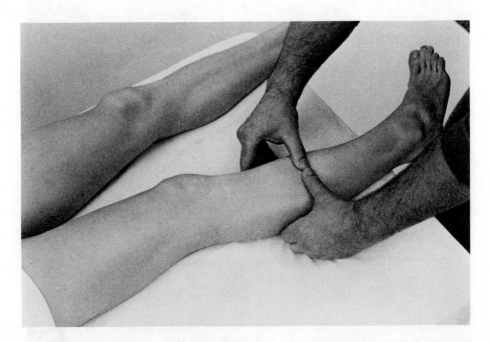

Deep Stroking of the Lower Leg Turn the athlete's foot slightly inward to make the muscles of the outer shin more accessible. Then, with the thumbs tip to tip and the hands on either side of the calf, deep-stroke the length of the muscle on the outside of the shin from the ankle to (but not including) the knee. Repeat this movement at least three times.

Do not deep-stroke the inside of the shin. When worked from the front, the fine, hairlike tendons which attach the inner shin (gastrocnemius) to the back of the tibia sometimes become inflamed. This area is best worked from the back.

Conclude the massage with some light strokes and repeat these movements on the other leg.

Back of the Leg

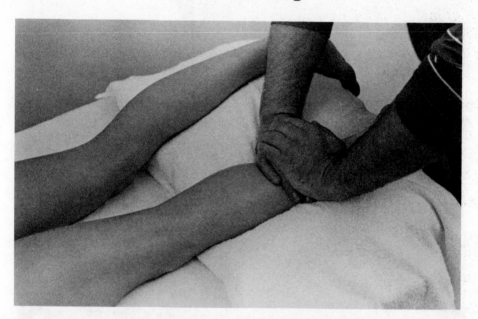

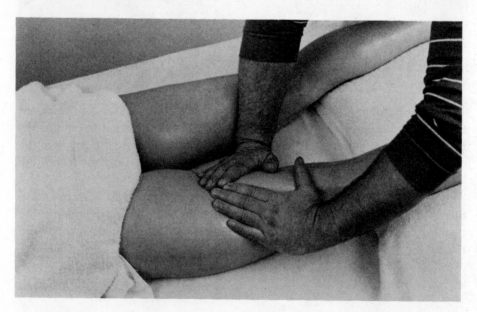

Light Stroking of the Back of the Leg   With the athlete lying face down, stand next to his feet and stroke gently with your hands flat from the calf to the buttock. Glide the hands back and repeat the movement at least four times. This stroke warms the area, preparing it for the other movements.

Uncomfortable pressure can be taken off the knees by resting the shins on a thick pillow.

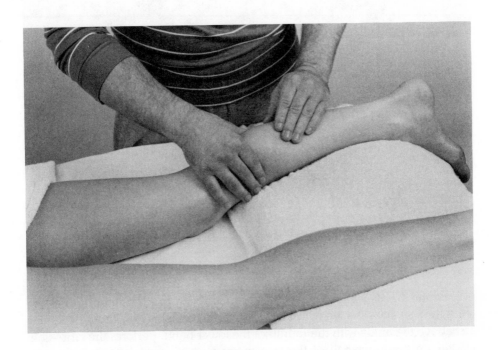

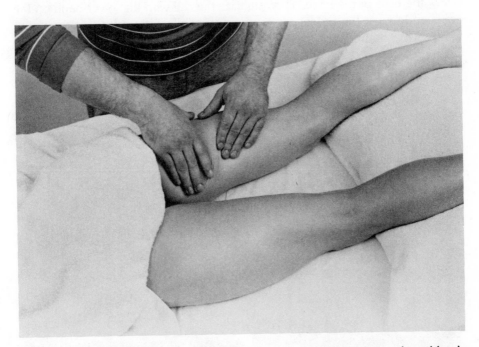

Kneading of the Back of the Leg From a position next to the athlete's knee, begin kneading the inside of the leg from the calf to the buttock and back. Repeat at least three times, making sure to cover the entire back of the leg.

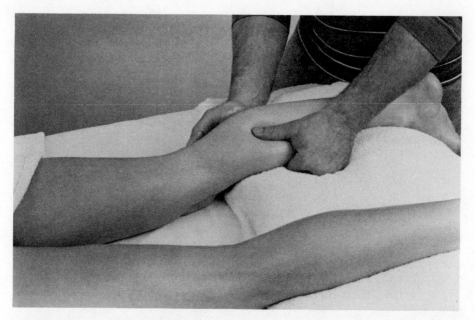

Broad Cross-Fiber Stroking of the Calf From a position by the athlete's foot, stabilize the leg with the upper hand just below the knee. Beginning just above the ankle with the thumb of the lower hand, perform the cross-fiber strokes on the inner half of the calf, moving up in overlapping rows to just below the base of the knee. Then stabilize the calf with the lower hand on the ankle and repeat the procedure on the outer half of the calf using the upper hand. Cover both inner and outer calf three times.

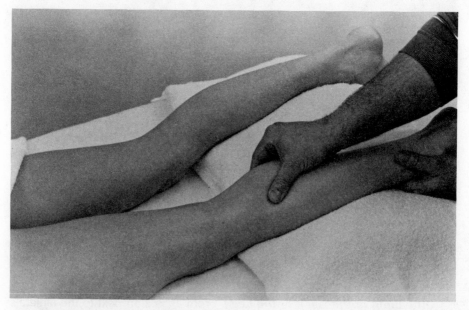

Jostling the Calf Loosely grasp the calf muscle just below the knee and shake it back and forth as you move down to the ankle. Repeat at least three times.

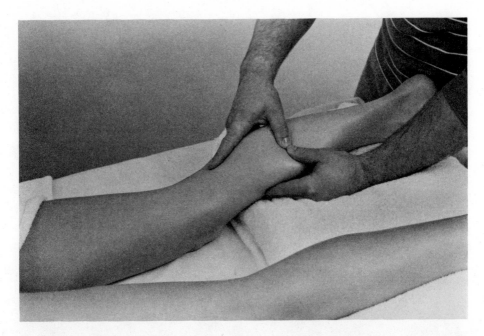

Deep Stroking of the Calf From a position beneath the foot, place fingertips on either side of calf and deep-stroke it with the thumbs. Begin just above the Achilles tendon and end just below the knee so as to avoid irritating tendons. Cover the entire calf with these strokes. Repeat at least three times.

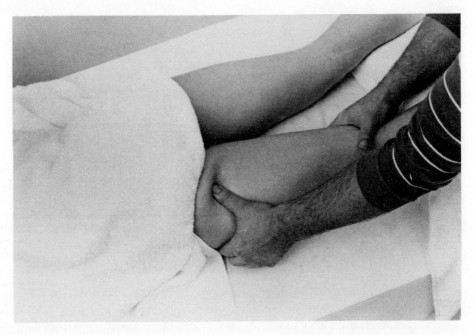

Broad Cross-Fiber Stroking of the First Section (Iliotibial Band) In your mind, divide the back of the athlete's thigh into four sections, running lengthwise from the hip to the knee. From a position next to the athlete's legs, stabilize the knee with the lower hand, grasping the inside of the knee firmly. Use the thumb of the upper hand to cross-stroke the outer edge of the leg, from the buttock to just above the knee and back up again. Repeat this movement at least three times.

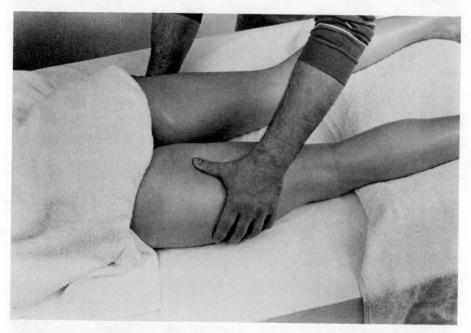

Broad Cross-Fiber Stroking of the Second Section (Biceps Femoris) The second section is adjacent to the first. Begin at the buttock and perform cross-fiber strokes of this section, overlapping the first section and stroking to just above the knee. Stroke the length of the section and back again. Repeat the movement at least three times.

Stroke the remaining two sections on the other side of the leg, following the same procedure as for sections one and two.

Jostling of the Back of the Upper Leg (See facing page above.) With the upper hand stabilizing the outside of the thigh, loosely grasp the flesh in each section with the lower hand, shaking it vigorously for about five seconds and then proceeding to the next quadrant. Jostle the back of the upper leg three times.

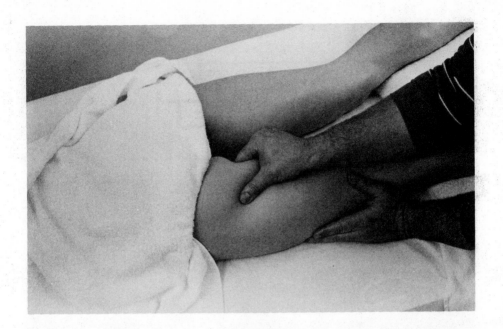

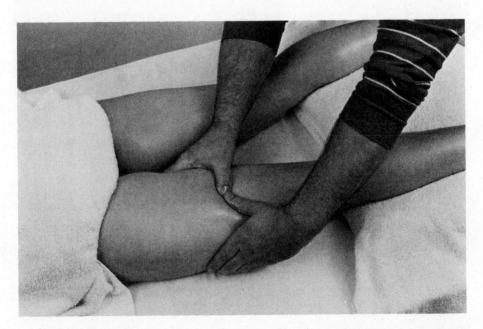

Deep Stroking of the Sections From a position next to the athlete's legs, place the fingers on either side of the thigh and deep-stroke the individual sections with the joined thumbs, applying pressure on the strokes toward the buttock and gliding back down. Be sure to cover the entire section with strokes before proceeding to the next section. Repeat the movements at leat three times on each section, except the outermost section, the iliotibial band. This is tendon, and shouldn't be deep-stroked.

Finish the massage with light stroking of the entire leg. Repeat the procedure on the other leg.

9 · FEET

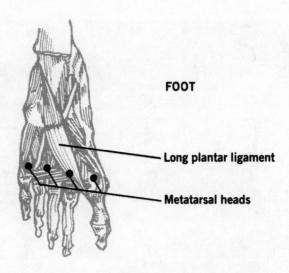

FOOT

Long plantar ligament

Metatarsal heads

Highly complex, the foot is made up of twenty-six separate bones connected by ligaments and controlled by dozens of muscles. Because of its anatomical complexity, it is easily injured. Due to the large number of tendons and ligaments, sprains are the most common injury. A sprained foot or ankle is an injury of these tissues. Tendons and ligaments can be kept pliable with frequent preventive massage.

Preventive massage can also make the muscles of the feet more pliable and less likely to tear. This is important in an area of the body where several small muscles undergo extreme stress.

In addition to the ligaments and muscles, the foot contains many important tendons, those fibrous strings that attach muscle to bone. Among them is that rope of a tendon, the Achilles, which runs up the back of the foot, connecting the calf to the heel.

Tendons don't shorten with exercise; however, the muscles they attach to do shorten, causing the tendons to pull and sometimes tear at the muscle or bone attachment. Sometimes the pulling can irritate the tendon inside its sheath, creating swelling and scar tissue. The value of massage is that it lengthens the muscles that pull on the tendons, relieving the strain.

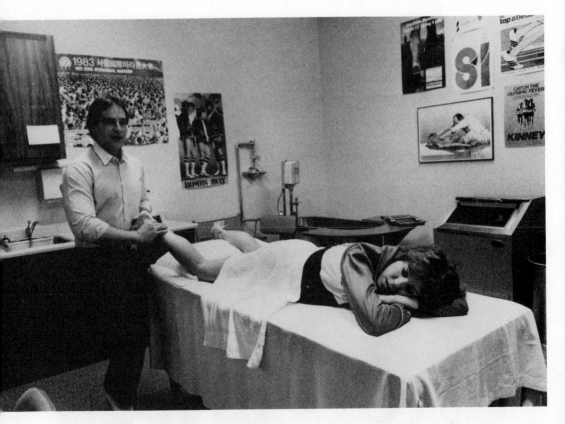

Preparing the Foot Facing the foot, stabilize it by placing the upper hand on the top of the foot. Take the heel of the other hand and run it up and down the bottom of the foot. Use a lot of pressure, since the feet can withstand more pressure than most areas of the body. This movement is called "warming the foot" because it does just that, increasing the blood flow for the upcoming strokes.

There are many types of tendinitis, including Achilles tendinitis; extensor tendinitis, which is strain of the tendon that runs down the top of the foot directly into the toes; and posterior tibial tendinitis, which occurs on the bottom of the foot and affects the tendon that supports the arch. The plantar fascia, a broad band of connective tissue on the bottom of the foot, is a frequent source of pain and inflammation beneath the heelbone, especially among distance runners. Keeping the plantar fascia flexible and the muscles of the arch loose greatly diminishes the risks of this injury.

Foot health is important to almost every sport. When muscles or tendons become tight or are injured, the athlete's running style is altered, which puts stress on muscles not ordinarily exposed to it. The result can be a chain reaction of injury that moves up the leg, sometimes as far as the back. It is the athletic version of the domino theory.

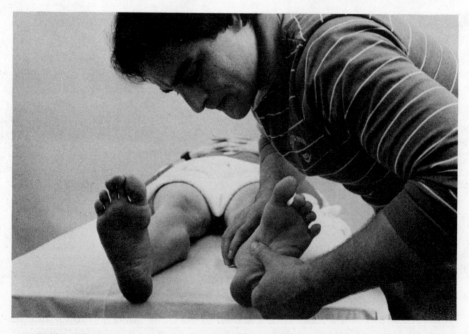

Deep Stroking of the Arch and Heel   With the upper hand on top of the athlete's foot, begin stroking the length of the arch and heel with the thumb of the lower hand, working from the inside of the foot to the outside and back again. Repeat at least four times.

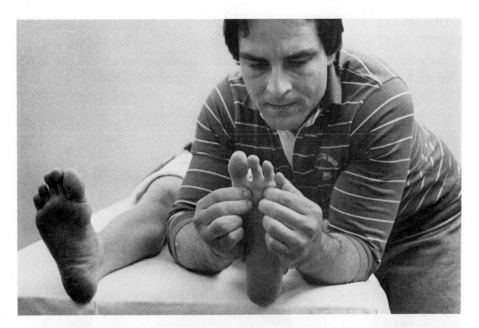

Deep Stroking Between the Metatarsal Heads Turning your body so you face the top of the foot and resting your arms on the table, place your fingers between the athlete's metatarsals—bones located in the middle part of the foot—and stroke toward the heel with the fingertips. Apply a great deal of pressure, stroking down to the arch. Repeat at least four times.

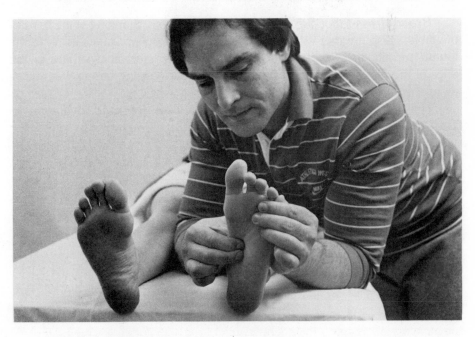

Broad Cross-Fiber Stroking of the Lower Foot Stabilizing the foot with a firm grip on the metatarsals, cross the foot in rows from the heel to the metatarsals and back again. You can use either the fingers or the thumb to execute these strokes. Repeat this movement at least four times.

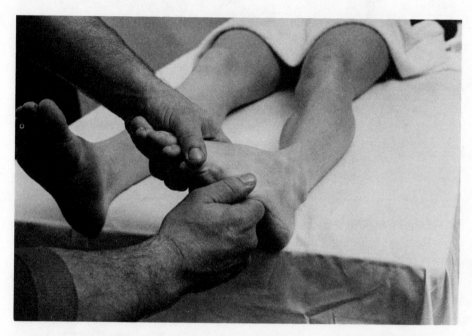

Broad Cross-Fiber Stroking of the Outer Foot   Standing at the base of the table, grasp the foot with the inside hand across the metatarsals. With the thumb and fingers of the outside hand, administer cross-fiber strokes to the edge of the foot from the toes to the heel and back again. Repeat that movement at least five times.

Finish the foot massage with the same strokes you used to prepare it. Then repeat the series on the other foot.

10 · BUTTOCKS

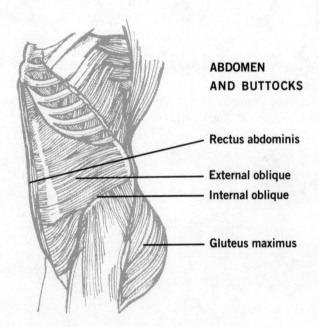

ABDOMEN AND BUTTOCKS

Rectus abdominis

External oblique

Internal oblique

Gluteus maximus

This is the location of the sprinter's power; broad, thick and fleshy muscles responsible in part for explosiveness and also for our ability to stand erect.

Because of their mass and the fact that unlike most muscles they rarely stretch to their limit, the buttocks muscles don't experience the microtears in the muscle fibers that other muscles do.

However, they do at times become extremely sore from lactic acid that builds up during exercise, and they are prone to spasm from prolonged exertion. They also tighten in sympathy to hamstring and lower back strain. Hence, preventive massage for the buttocks must remove the bad chemicals of exercise from the muscles, freshening them with increased blood supply. Massage also keeps the muscles of this area loose and pliable.

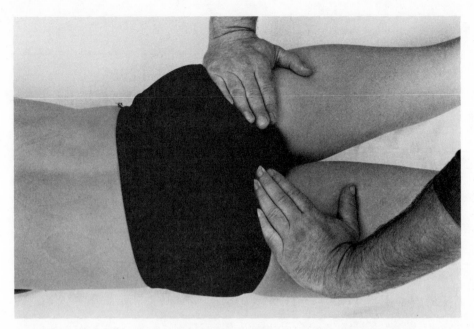

Light Stroking of the Buttocks From a position next to the athlete's upper legs, use the palms and fingers of each hand to stroke the muscles of the buttocks, from the "cheeks" to the lower back. Repeat this at least four times to prepare the muscles for the deeper strokes.

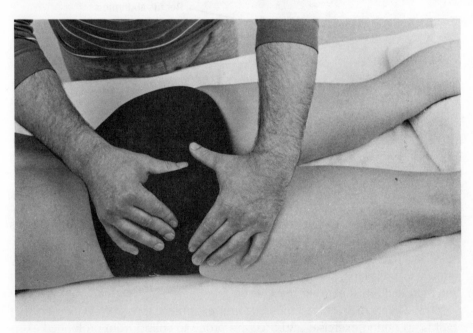

Kneading of the Buttocks Standing next to the athlete's buttocks, reach across and grasp the buttock farthest away. Knead it from the upper leg to the lower back, making sure to cover the entire muscle, from the midline to the outer edge. Repeat at least three times before doing the other side.

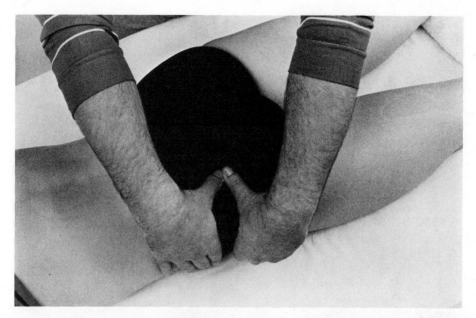

Broad Cross-Fiber Stroking of the Buttocks Reach across the buttocks and hold your thumbs side by side so they point toward you. Push the thumbs into the flesh and pull them across the buttock. Start at the cheek and move up in rows to the crest of the lower back. Repeat at least three times before doing the other side.

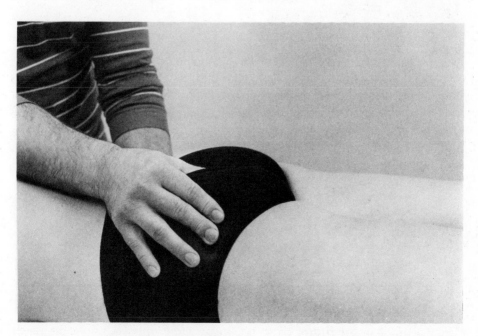

Jostling of the Buttocks Standing next to the athlete's lower back, grasp the far buttock between your thumb and fingers and jostle vigorously for about five seconds. Repeat at least three times before doing the other side.

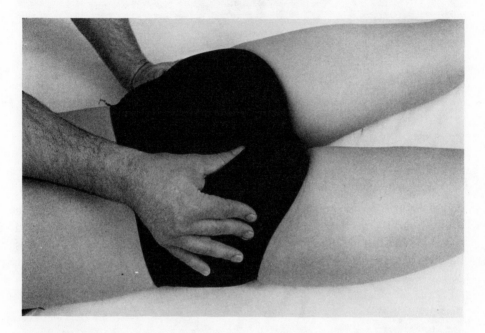

Deep Stroking of the Buttocks Standing next to the buttocks, reach across the athlete and deep-stroke the far buttock. Deep strokes run parallel to the alignment of muscle, so these strokes should be done with the thumb of one hand pushing down at a forty-five-degree angle from the spine toward the cheek. Cover the entire muscle, with rows of strokes from the midline of the buttocks to the hip. Repeat three times before doing the other side.

Conclude the massage with several light strokes of the buttocks.

11 · BACK

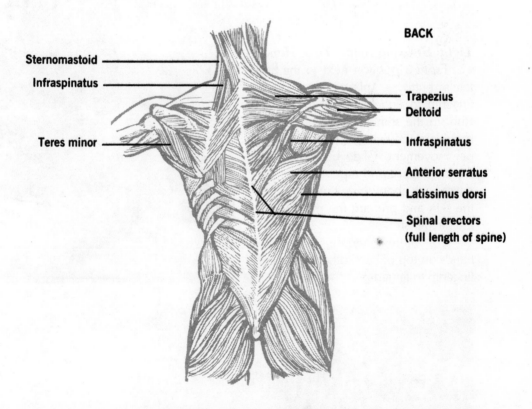

BACK

Sternomastoid

Infraspinatus

Teres minor

Trapezius

Deltoid

Infraspinatus

Anterior serratus

Latissimus dorsi

Spinal erectors
(full length of spine)

A comfortable back—free of muscle tightness, pains and strains—is as necessary as it is difficult to achieve. Every sport, from running to rowing, requires a
healthy back.

But the back seldom cooperates. Like a machine with many moving parts,
something is always breaking down. In preventive massage, we try to maintain
the balance of the muscles of the back to prevent these breakdowns.

Some of the muscles we are primarily concerned with are the latissimus dorsi, the spinal erectors and the muscles over the shoulder blades.

The latissimus dorsi muscles, or "lats," run down the sides of the back from beneath the armpit and are the main pulling muscles used in such activities as rowing or chin-ups.

The spinal erectors are small muscles providing stability to the vertebrae. They keep the spine aligned and are subject to stress in almost any sport.

Like the lats, the muscles over the shoulder blades are also pulling muscles, subject to stress in sports that require pulling or throwing.

Light Stroking with Two Hands

From a position next to the athlete's buttocks, place your hands fingertip to fingertip over the spine. Rub up the spine all the way to the shoulders, covering about one foot per movement. Glide back down to the lower back and repeat. Cover the entire back about three times to warm the skin and prepare the muscles for the deeper strokes.

For more pressure, place the hands on top of each other instead of fingertip to fingertip.

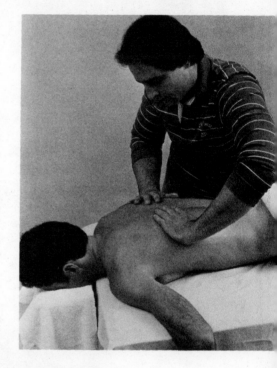

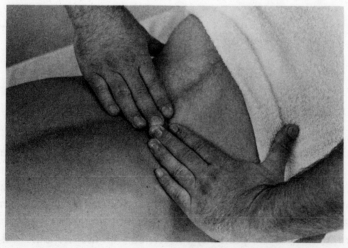

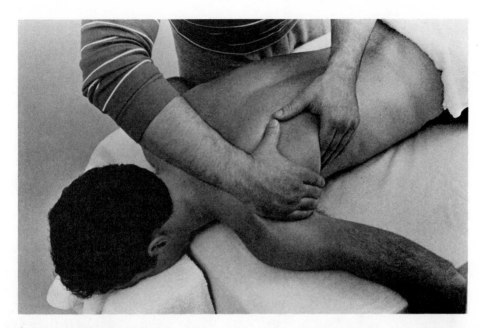

Kneading of the Sides of the Back (Latissimus Dorsi) The muscles that run down the sides of the back, from the armpit almost to the base of the rib cage, are the latissimus dorsi muscles. From a position next to the middle of the athlete's back, reach across and grasp the far lat with both hands, kneading it with alternate strokes of the hands from under the armpit to the hip and back again. Repeat this movement three times on each side of the back. This will further relax the muscles and create a stronger hyperemia.

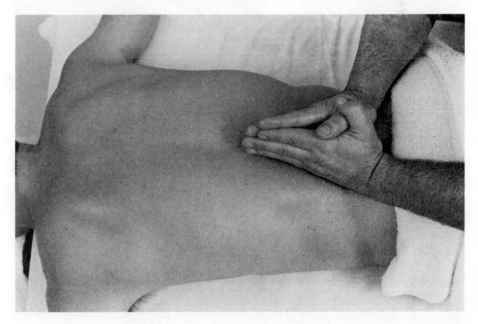

Fanning of the Back From a position next to the athlete's buttocks, hold the hands prayer fashion on the lower spine. Push the hands down and

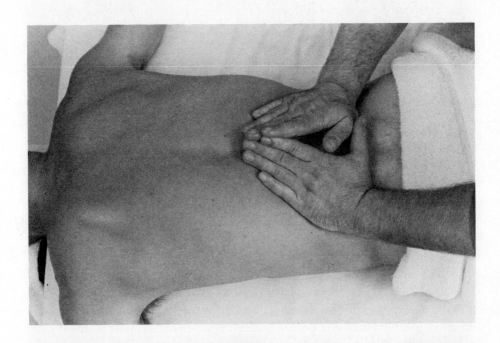

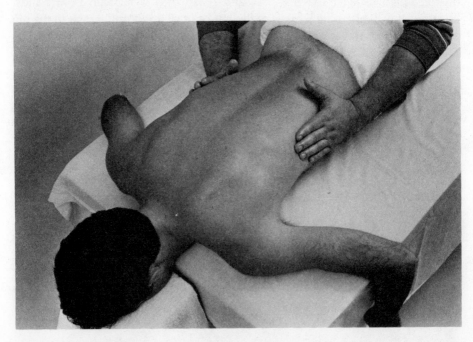

spread them out, applying pressure to the back with the sides of your hands and palms. When returning to the spine, lift the sides of the abdomen with your fingertips, keeping contact with the athlete's skin. Repeat this movement at least three times before moving your hands up to cover the next hand-length. Cover the entire back all the way to the shoulders.

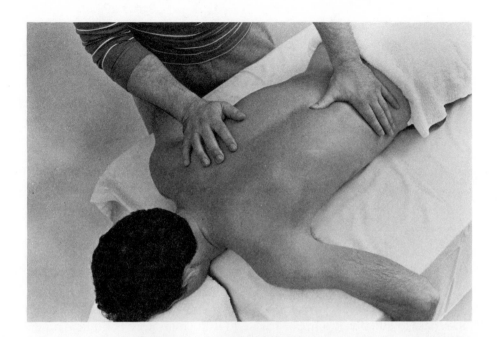

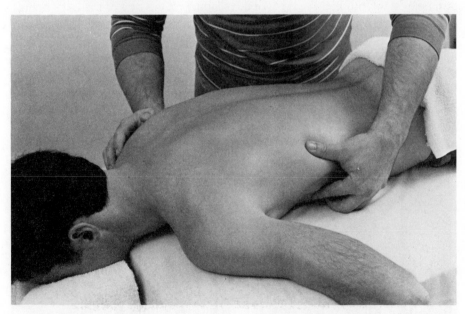

Broad Cross-Fiber Stroking of the Outside of the Back   From next to
the middle of the athlete's back, and with your upper hand on the upper back
for stability, place the thumb of your lower hand just across the spine at the
lower back. Push away from the spine with the thumb, using deep pressure all
the way to the edge of the back. Move row by row up the side of the spine,
making sure that your strokes overlap slightly. When you reach the shoulder
blade, shorten the strokes so you don't hit the bone. Cover this side of the
back at least three times before performing the same movements on the other
side.

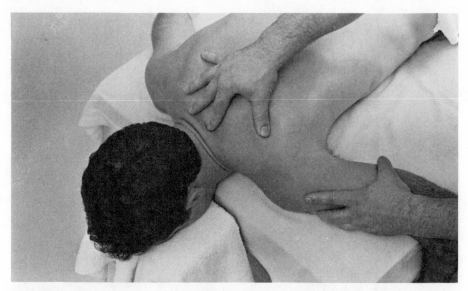

Broad Cross-Fiber Stroking Over the Shoulder Blade (Scapula)
From next to the athlete's upper back and with your upper hand holding the arm nearest to you, find the base of the scapula on the side of the back nearest to you. It is almost even with the armpit. With your fingers extending up toward the base of the neck, push the thumb across the scapula upward, at a forty-five-degree angle to the spine. The last inch of this stroke will also cover the trapezius, the muscles on either side of the neck. Stroke in rows beginning near the spine and moving out to the end of the shoulder. Repeat at least three times before performing these movements on the other scapula.

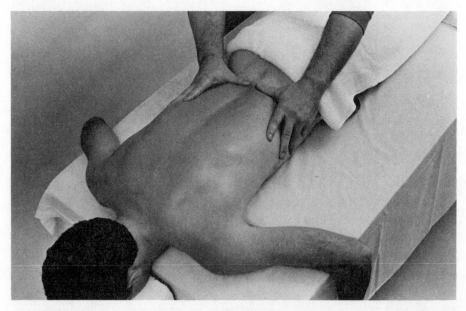

Deep Stroking of the Spine Muscles (Spinal Erectors)   On either side of the spine are the spinal erector muscles, which provide much of the spine's stability. From a position next to the athlete's buttocks, place your thumbs on either side of the spine near the small of the back. Stroke slowly and deeply with both thumbs, instructing the athlete to breathe slowly and deeply as your thumbs progress up the spine a few inches at a time. Cover the entire spine all the way to the shoulders at least three times, rubbing progressively deeper each time.

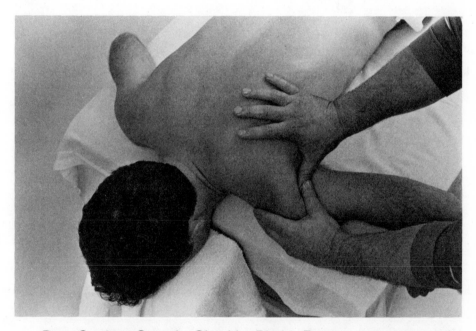

Deep Stroking Over the Shoulder Blade   From a position next to the athlete's shoulder, place one thumb over the other on the base of the scapula closest to you. Push toward the spine, beginning at the base of the scapula and working in rows up to the base of the trapezius. Cover the area at least three times before repeating the movements on the other shoulder blade.

Complete the back massage with general light stroking with the palms.

12 · NECK

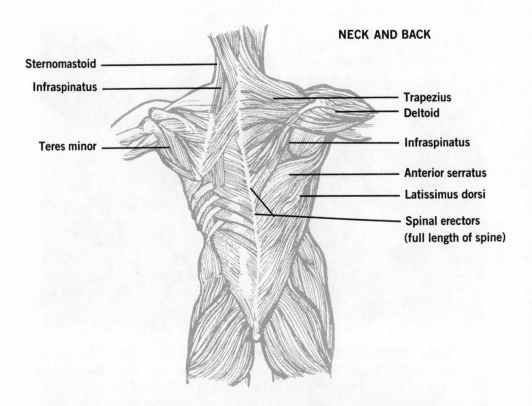

NECK AND BACK

Sternomastoid

Infraspinatus

Teres minor

Trapezius

Deltoid

Infraspinatus

Anterior serratus

Latissimus dorsi

Spinal erectors
(full length of spine)

The diversity of the neck, with its ability to twist and bend to many angles, is also its downfall. Even a sport like distance running, which doesn't seem to involve the neck, can cause tension in this area.

In preventive massage, we perform movements to stretch the muscles of the cervical spine, those seven vertebrae that make up the neck.

We also concentrate upon the larger support muscles, such as the formidable sternocleidomastoids, which run down the sides of the neck and provide much of the neck's ability to twist. Also important are the trapezius muscles on top of the shoulders, which provide support and power.

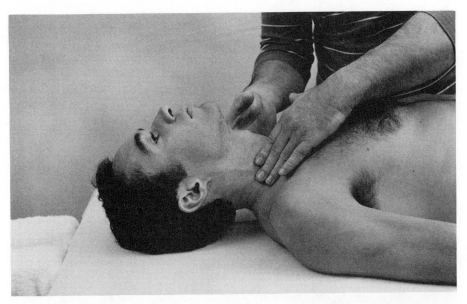

Light Stroking of the Neck With the athlete on his back, arms at his sides, stroke gently with the fingertips across the back of the shoulders to the base of the skull. Use both hands at the same time, on both sides of the neck. Repeat at least three times, each stroke slightly deeper than the one before.

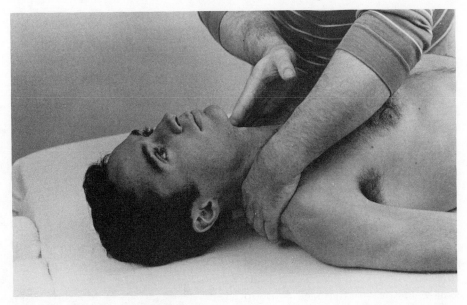

Kneading of the Neck and Trapezius Placing your hands on the athlete's shoulders, knead the trapezius muscles to the base of the neck with both hands. Then knead the muscles with the circular motion of petrissage. Work up the back of the neck to the base of the skull with the petrissage movement. Repeat this sequence at least three times.

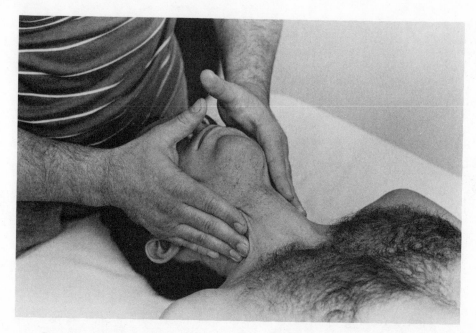

Petrissage of the Side of the Neck (Sternocleidomastoid) Standing directly above and behind the athlete, put your fingertips on the long muscles that are easily felt on either side of the neck, beginning directly below the ears. Rub in a slow, circular fashion (petrissage) until you have covered the entire muscle, from the base of the ear to the collarbone. Repeat at least three times.

Broad Cross-Fiber Stroking of the Side of the Neck Cradle the athlete's head in one hand and turn it to the side. With the thumb of the free hand, cross the side of the neck in rows, moving from the base of the skull to the base of the neck. Perform these strokes slowly. Rapid movements can be painful and can cause tension in the athlete's neck. Repeat this movement at least three times on both sides of the neck.

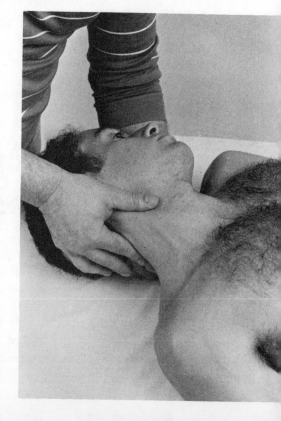

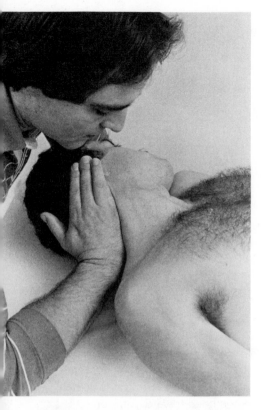

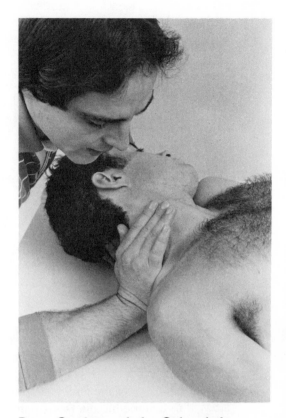

Blading of the Neck and the Trapezius Cradling the athlete's head with the palm of one hand, turn it so the cheek is up. Place the edge of your hand beneath the base of the ear and stroke slowly down the side of the neck and the trapezius. Perform this movement gently at first and then progressively deeper. Repeat at least three times, then do the other side of the neck.

Deep Stroking of the Side of the Neck with the Fingertips With the athlete's head cradled and the cheek up, deep-stroke the side of the neck with your fingertips, moving in a straight line from the base of the skull to the base of the neck. Make sure you cover the entire muscle, increasing pressure slightly with each pass. Since it is a narrow muscle, two passes will cover it. Repeat the movement at least three times before doing the other side of the neck.

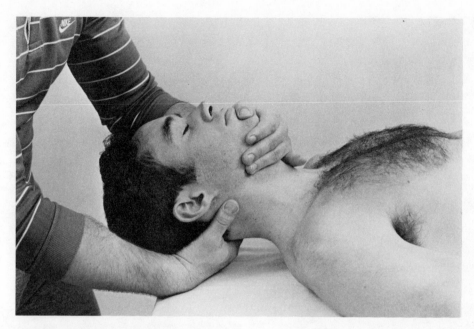

Neck Pull   In this movement it is important that the athlete clasp his hands over his navel and leave his legs uncrossed so the muscles of the spine don't become twisted. Place your right hand under the base of the skull and the left hand under the jaw. Have the athlete take a deep breath and exhale slowly through the mouth. As he exhales, pull the head toward you, firmly but not hard. Remind the athlete to relax as you pull. Repeat at least three times.

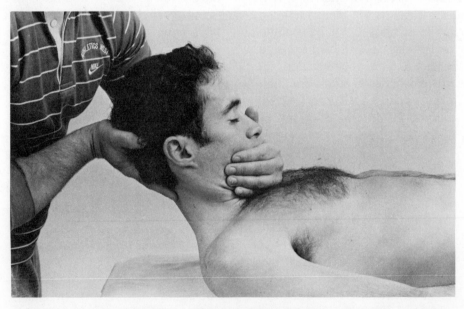

Neck Stretch   Change the position of your right hand so that the finger-tips extend down toward the neck. Place the left hand across the chin and mouth. Have the athlete take another deep breath and exhale slowly. As he exhales, lift the head slightly, dropping the chin slowly toward the chest until the exhalation ends. Then lower the head to the table and repeat with another exhale. Repeat this movement at least three times.

Have the athlete turn over onto his stomach.

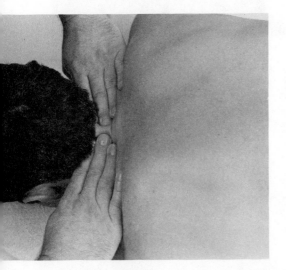

Light Stroking of the Neck and Shoulders Positioning yourself at the athlete's head, stroke firmly with the fingertips (not the palms) from the base of the skull to the shoulders. Thoroughly cover the neck and the trapezius at least three times.

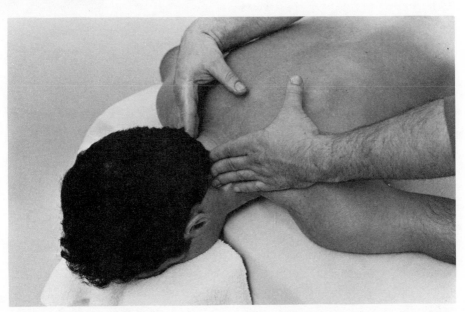

Petrissage of the Neck and Shoulders Standing next to the athlete, administer the circular strokes of petrissage from the base of the skull to the base of the neck. This will serve to further loosen the muscles of the neck and shoulders. Repeat at least three times.

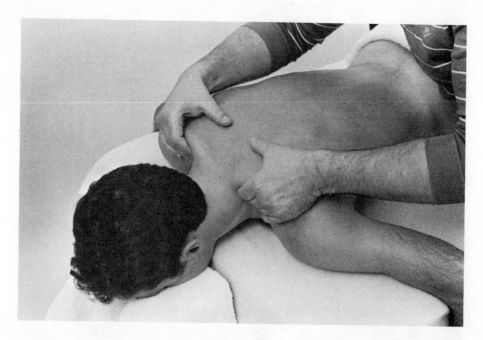

Kneading of the Trapezius Grasp the trapezius between the thumb and fingers, kneading the muscle to the base of the neck and back. Repeat at least three times.

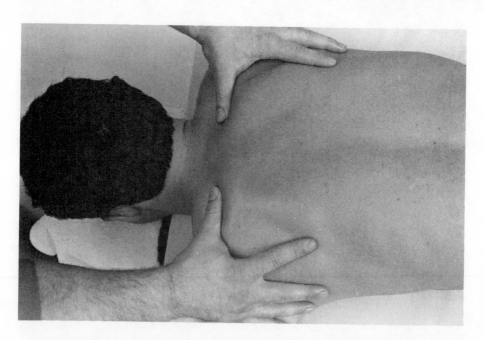

Broad Cross-Fiber Stroking of the Trapezius Standing at the athlete's head, place your thumbs on the trapezius on either side of the neck and push them straight down to the base of the muscle. Move out in rows to the ends of the trapezius. Repeat at least three times.

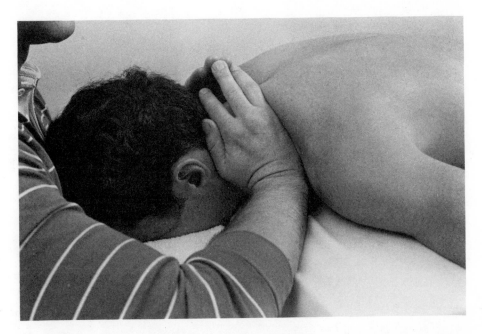

Blading of the Trapezius Place the edge of your hands on the sides of the athlete's neck at the base of the skull. Push into the flesh, maintaining constant pressure as you push the hands down the neck and along the trapezius to the shoulder. Repeat this stroke at least three times.

Complete the massage with some light stroking of the neck and shoulders.

PART THREE

CURATIVE MASSAGE

13 · INTRODUCTION

When I was in private practice, I had many chronically injured patients. I have also had many since then, but even compared to them, one from my days in private practice was exceptional.

On one visit he would come in complaining about a strain to his shoulder caused by a racquetball game that he didn't warm up for properly.

Another time he would come in with a torn Achilles tendon or strained hamstring from running too much or too hard.

Sometimes fate—in the form of a 200-pound rugby player—would deal him a cruel blow on a local playing field. He would come in limping from a blind-side hit to the knee or even a traumatic injury to the chest from a collision.

I used to call him a car wreck waiting to happen. He called himself a hard-charging athlete. I suspect we were both right. Although he had more than his share of injuries, he was a weekend athlete who loved to test himself. As he put it: "The only way to keep yourself from getting injured is to stay out of the arena of competiton. I would be bored if I did that."

Most of us would. Although we don't like injuries, as athletes we have learned to accept a certain number of them. And, of course, we have learned a variety of ways to cope with them.

For most of you, curative massage will be a new way of dealing with those injuries. It can do more to heal and nourish damaged muscular and connective tissue than any other form of therapy. Not only does it improve blood circulation to the injured area, it aligns the torn fibers so scar tissue can form parallel to muscle fibers in a way that won't cause the irregular, thick and weak scarring that creates muscle spasm.

Mary Decker's calves were among the worst examples of improperly healed tears that I have ever seen. Her calves were injured repeatedly during her early years (ages eleven to twenty). Not being the sort to rest much, she never gave the tears a chance to heal evenly. When I began treating her in 1980, Mary's calves felt like a sack of marbles.

It was my slow and painstaking task to soften that scar tissue, massaging it so deeply that the body's fluids would permeate the scar tissue and soften it.

That's another curative aspect of massage. Done properly, it can remove the lumpiness by creating an improved circulation, or fibrovascular network, in the scar tissue.

This makes the scar tissue more pliable and less likely to tear. It also makes it less like a callous and more like skin, which means it won't irritate surrounding tissue, causing spasm.

Curative massage is usually left to the professional, perhaps because most people feel they will do more damage than good in applying it. As you may have guessed, I don't agree with that.

There is very little that a person can do to cause muscle damage with massage. Occasionally, a deep massage will cause bruising, usually because small blood vessels beneath scar tissue are broken. Although this is rare, don't let an infrequent bruise deter you from your efforts. When bruises appear, it is because the tissue is not pliable. This is an area in need of massage.

Nor is soreness to the area a day or two after the massage a rare occurrence. This is normal in a deeply massaged area. It means that the athlete should reduce his training if the injury hasn't already caused him to slow down or lay off.

Of course, curative massage must be properly performed to be valuable. I have identified eight rules to follow in curative massage. You should familiarize yourself with these rules before plunging thumbs first into any of these movements.

• *If an athlete is resting or in limited training, use curative massage every day, sometimes even twice a day.* In these cases, the injury is usually bad enough that it requires the tissue to be freed of inflammation and tension as often as possible.

• *If the athlete is continuing to train, use these techniques only on days of easy workouts.* Here the injury is not severe enough to stop training and therefore requires less attention.

• *Use synchronized breathing techniques whenever possible.* Have the athlete breathe deeply and rhythmically. Stroke on the out breaths. Not only will this help the athlete relax, it will also increase the depth and effectiveness of the strokes.

• *Never use deep strokes parallel to long tendons or ligaments.* Long tendons with sheaths, such as the Achilles tendon, are highly susceptible to inflammation when stroked along their length. Also, in the case of a strained Achilles, parallel deep strokes can worsen the tear.

● *Treat newly injured areas gently.* I advise not massaging the area for as long as forty-eight hours after an injury or until the swelling has gone down. Little can be accomplished with massage during this period anyway, since the area is usually filled with blood and fluid.

● *If treating specific areas of spasm or scar tissue, use mainly local cross-fiber stroking.* This stroke allows you to put the emphasis where it is needed, on fibers that must be spread out.

● *If the athlete begins to resist or becomes tense, ask him to relax and jostle the area.* Relaxation is important to effective massage because it is easier to manipulate tissue when it is relaxed. If you feel the athlete tense up from the manipulation of a tender area, stop and lightly jostle the muscle. Also have him concentrate on relaxation. Synchronized breathing will help.

● *Work deeply, not sadistically.* It is necessary to work as deeply as the athlete's tolerance will permit in performing curative massage. However, don't plunge right in at first to the depths of the muscle. Proceed slowly, remembering that the athlete's tolerance will increase as the area is worked and the pain and tension subside.

Three strokes accomplish most of the work in curative massage. Although these are covered in detail in Chapter 3, "Methods of Massage," I'll cover them again briefly here:

● *Deep strokes:* These are usually applied with the thumbs, pushing parallel to the length of the muscles, spreading the muscle fibers along the way.

You will often find "knots" as you administer deep strokes. These knots feel like tiny spheres of hard tissue, like those marbles I mentioned in Mary Decker's calves. Deep stroking is the most productive movement in the elimination of these problem areas. It helps smooth the spasmed muscle and enhances the flow of blood and lymph to the area.

● *Broad cross-fiber strokes:* Like deep strokes, these strokes are familiar from preventive massage. Usually performed with the thumb, they cross the muscle, pulling the muscle fibers apart so they don't stick together.

When broad cross-fiber strokes are applied, the muscle should not snap back like a taut rope. If it does, you have located a problem area. If an entire muscle snaps back when released, you have found a muscle in general spasm. If the area that snaps back is small and does not cover the entire length of the muscle, you have probably found an area injured in the past where the fibers still cling to one another.

● *Local cross-fiber strokes:* These are used only in curative massage.

These strokes should be applied with the fingertips or thumb. Wipe the oil off the skin to give you greater control of the tissue. Unlike other strokes, your fingers won't move over the skin. Instead, you will manipulate the skin to cross the fibers of a specific area very deeply.

Don't worry about applying too much pressure unless the injury is acute and light pressure brings pain. If that happens, use these strokes gently for the purpose of reducing inflammation.

Local cross-fiber strokes work directly on the injured area. Their effect is almost like reweaving the muscle fibers together so the scar tissue can form with less irritation to the surrounding area.

I have spent as long as forty-five minutes applying local cross-fiber strokes to one tendon. Generally, however, anything over fifteen minutes is not especially valuable. You will notice that most of the following routines call for just a few minutes of local cross-fiber strokes, which is enough to make a tremendous change in the condition of the injury.

Each sport has a unique set of motions, which means that certain muscles are more likely to be injured than others. The following is a list of sports and the areas most likely to be injured by the stresses of the sport. This list does not include traumatic injuries that can result anywhere on the body from contact with other athletes or the playing surface.

• *Running:* As you may have guessed, most of the injuries in running happen to the feet and legs. Plantar fascitis, which is an inflammation of a tendon on the bottom of the foot, is the most common foot injury. Achilles tendinitis is a frequent and sometimes debilitating injury, as are shin splints, which are less serious but sometimes just as annoying. The sport even has an injury named for it: "runner's knee," or chondromalacia, which is an irritation of the tendons under the kneecap.

Because running is the act of propelling the body forward, the muscles in the back of the legs receive the brunt of the strain, particularly the hamstrings, from which runners seem to suffer an inordinate amount of grief. Because of this propelling action, the sciatic nerve also has a tendency to become irritated.

• *Racquet sports:* The explosiveness of these sports and the likelihood of improper warm-up makes the player susceptible to shoulder and elbow tendinitis, commonly known as "tennis elbow."

• *Cycling:* The lower back and the neck are two areas likely to be in need of curative massage, because they are locked when the cyclist is in position. The bicycle's propulsion system—the legs—may also need curative attention, especially the hamstrings and quadriceps.

• *Basketball:* Contact injuries aside, the most likely problems will result from knee and ankle tendinitis caused by the repeated cutting and jumping on the hard playing surface.

• *Swimming:* If anything is injured in this sport, it will probably be the shoulders, due to the rotation of the arms. The upper back often suffers some chronic tightness from the constant windmill action of the arms.

- *Skiing:* Thigh and knee strain are prevalent in skiing, due not only to the ruggedness of the sport but also to the athlete's failure to warm up properly before charging down the slopes.
- *Golf:* Yes, even golf has its injuries, mainly to the lower back from holding a bent-over position and twisting.
- *Soccer:* Leg injuries are most common in this sport. The groin, ankles and knees are likely to be injured from the quick changes in direction a player is forced to make.
- *Baseball:* The throwing of the ball and swinging of the bat can cause injury to the shoulders and upper back, but all of the other aspects of the Great American Sport tax the legs in every way imaginable.
- *Volleyball:* If play is done on a hard surface, the athlete may have shin splints to contend with from contact with the court and the repeated explosive leaps required to play the game above the net.

You will notice that the following curative massage routines include manipulation of the specific area of injury as well as the area surrounding it. That is because the muscles surrounding an injury tighten to protect the area and relieve it of its workload. For instance, the muscles of the buttocks almost always tighten when the hamstrings are torn. This is good for the injured area, which needs to be shielded from further activity. But while it prevents further injury, it doesn't promote healing. This is something you have to do yourself. Massage of the surrounding area smoothes out the spasms, putting the tear back together for healing.

Before curative massage is administered to any part of the body, be sure to warm up the area with light strokes and kneading. Without these movements first, the deep movements of curative massage will not be as effective as they would if the area were relaxed.

These warm-up movements are included at the beginning of each curative routine. Be sure to perform them before beginning the deeper strokes.

Unlike preventive massage, treatment cannot be so easily scheduled for the curative routines. Preventive massage is for a fatigued but normal body. Curative massage, on the other hand, is designed to heal damaged tissue. Hence, the frequency with which the massage should be given depends entirely upon the degree of the injury.

There are two rules to follow in scheduling curative massage.

1. If the injury is severe enough to prevent an athlete from participating in his sport, perform curative massage daily or twice daily on the injured area.
2. If the injury only slows the athlete down but doesn't stop him, perform the curative routines every other day, making sure they are light workout days. Performing curative massage after a hard workout will only increase the stress to an injured area.

14 · ACHILLES TENDINITIS

There is almost no movement involving the foot that doesn't bring the Achilles tendon into play. As a result, this most often used tendon is also the most frequently injured tendon.

Many Achilles problems are due to lack of elasticity. Because of this, the tendon is prone to irritation and/or inflammation when the calf muscle to which it is attached pulls and shortens from exercise.

Achilles tendinitis develops in a slow fashion. In the early stages the tendon feels stiff and sore in the morning but becomes more limber as it is used. Although there is some pain, it usually isn't severe enough to keep the athlete from his normal exercise routine.

It is at this point that the athlete should stop exercising and treat the injury before it worsens. But since the pain isn't that bad, most athletes take the gamble and continue with their normal exercise routines. Most often, they lose that gamble and the injury worsens.

When that happens, the tendon continues to ache and swell, at which point normal exercise becomes almost impossible.

Once the athlete feels the stiffness and soreness of tendinitis in his Achilles tendon, he should stop exercising, apply ice two or three times a day for twenty minutes per session and follow this curative massage routine.

Warm-up

Before beginning the curative strokes on the Achilles, prepare the area with the following warm-up routine.

Light Stroking of the Lower Leg Have the athlete lie on his stomach. From a position by the athlete's foot, stroke the lower leg from the ankle to the knee with the palm of your hand. Glide the palm back and repeat the movement at least four times.

Kneading of the Lower Leg From a position next to the calves, reach across the athlete and knead the far calf, from the ankle to just below the knee and back again. Repeat at least three times, then begin the curative routine.

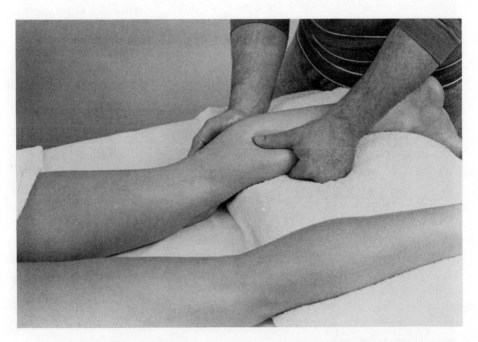

Broad Cross-Fiber Stroking of the Calf (Soleus) From next to the athlete's foot, stabilize the outside of the knee with your outside hand. With the thumb of the inside hand, cross the calf deeply in rows from just below the knee to just above the Achilles tendon. Repeat three times.

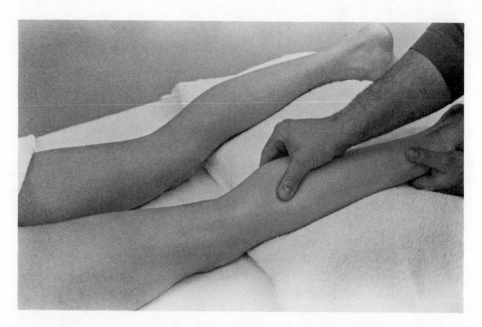

Jostling of the Calf From next to the athlete's foot, hold the ankle with the outside hand and grasp the calf with the thumb and fingers of the inside hand. Jostle the muscle for at least thirty seconds. Repeat three times, jostling at different places along the calf.

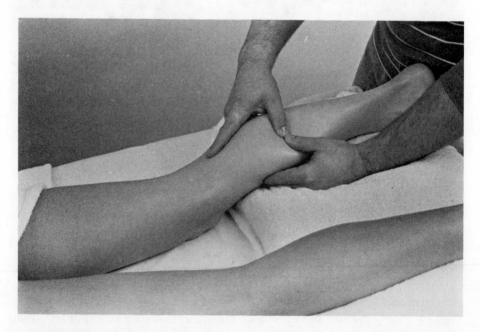

Deep Stroking of the Calf Place your fingers on either side of the athlete's calf and bring the tips of the thumbs together. Cover the entire calf with deep strokes from just above the Achilles tendon to just below the back of the knee. Repeat three times.

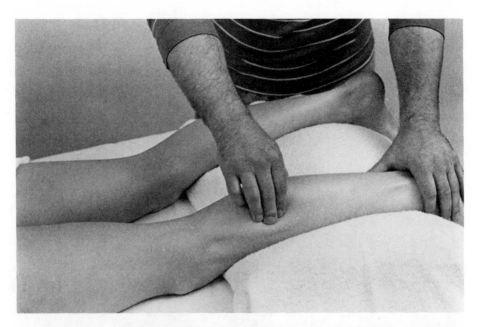

Local Cross-Fiber Stroking of the Calf Holding the ankle of the far leg with your lower hand, place your fingertips on the calf and administer local cross-fiber stroking. This loosens the calf along its attachment to the Achilles. Repeat at least three times.

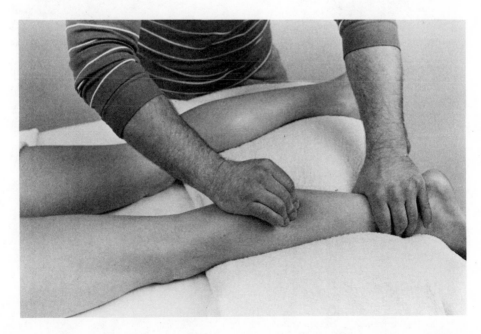

Local Cross-Fiber Stroking of the Calf at the Achilles Attachment Holding the ankle of the far leg with your lower hand, find the base of the calf with your fingertips. Apply local cross-fiber strokes as deeply as possible without causing discomfort. The strokes should last at least ten seconds and there should be no oil on the area being massaged. Repeat at least three times.

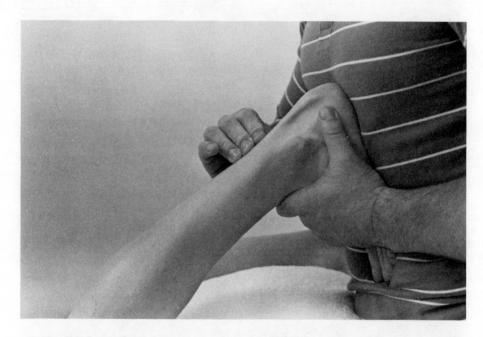

Local Cross-Fiber Stroking of the Stretched Achilles Tendon Lift the foot, propping it against your abdomen. This stretches the Achilles. Apply deep fingertip pressure back and forth across the tendon, starting at the heel attachment and working up to the attachment at the base of the calf. Work each tendon for at least five minutes.

This routine will loosen muscles that pull on the Achilles and will also break adhesions between the tendon and its sheath.

15 · LOWER BACK

All sports stress the lower back. This can cause muscle spasms in the area that places pressure on the nerves coming out of the spine, specifically the sciatic nerve. Some people suffer lower back stress more frequently than others. Why this is so is a source of medical disagreement. Some doctors claim that a misalignment of the hips causes a slight curvature of the lower spine, causing the muscles alongside it to spasm. Other doctors feel that muscular weaknesses in the abdomen and lower back cause surrounding muscles to spasm in an attempt to compensate for this weakness. Still others believe that a build-up of muscle tension is the sole culprit, and that relief of that tension through massage will allow the spine to straight itself out.

Whatever the cause, it has been my experience that lower back pain is most often eliminated by deep massage of the hamstring, buttocks muscles and all the other muscles that pull discontentedly at the lower back.

If you have a chronic lower backache that worsens after exercise, or one that won't allow you to exercise, perform the curative massage routine that follows. Do it once a day until the problem subsides. In addition to this routine, stretching exercises may be in order.

This massage will relax the muscles that may be applying pressure to the nerves that are irritating the lower back. It will also loosen the muscles that may be causing stiffness.

Thighs and Buttocks Warm-up

Before performing the curative movements, loosen the muscles of the area with the following massage routine.

Light Stroking of the Leg From a position by the shins, stroke the leg in one movement with the palms of the hands, from the knee to the buttock. Pressure should be firm but not deep during this stroke. Glide your hands back down and repeat the movement. This stroke should be done four times or until the athlete's skin becomes warm. Repeat on the other leg.

Kneading of the Leg From next to the athlete's thighs, knead the back of the thigh from the knee to the cheek of the buttock and back again. Make sure to cover the inside of the thigh as well as the back. These are large muscles and should be worked with considerable force. Cover the leg up and down at least three times. Repeat on the other leg.

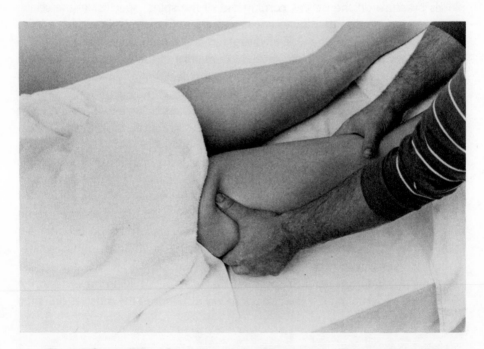

Broad Cross-Fiber Stroking of the Hamstring From next to the hip, reach across the athlete and administer broad cross-fiber strokes to the hamstring with the thumb of your lower hand. Strokes should cross the hamstring from just above the knee to the base of the buttock. Repeat three times.

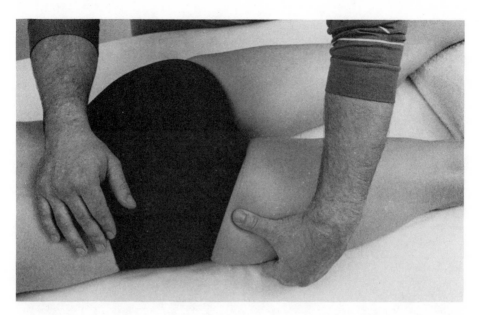

Broad Cross-Fiber Stroking of the Outside of the Thigh (Iliotibial Band) With your upper hand on the small of the athlete's back, reach across with your lower hand and administer broad cross-fiber strokes to the outside of the thigh with your thumb. Cover this area from the base of the buttock to just above the knee. Repeat three times.

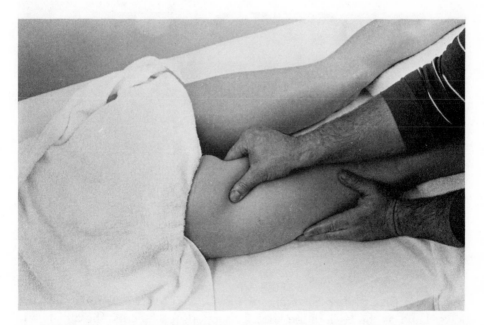

Jostling of the Hamstring From next to the shin of the leg you are massaging, grasp the athlete's hamstring with the thumb and fingers of your inside hand and jostle the muscle vigorously for at least thirty seconds. Repeat three times.

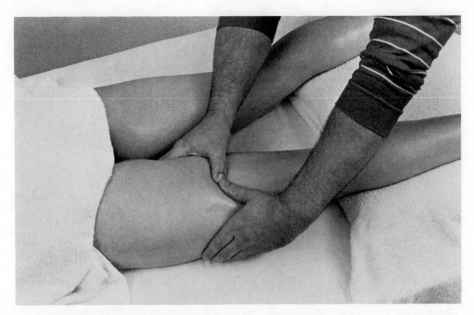

Deep Stroking of the Hamstring   With your fingers on both sides of the athlete's thigh, bring the tips of the thumbs together and administer deep strokes to the hamstring, covering the entire muscle in rows from just above the knee to the buttock. Repeat three times.

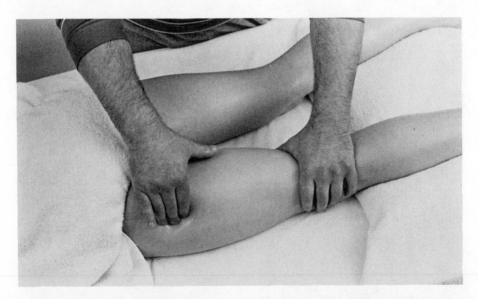

Local Cross-Fiber Stroking of the Outside of the Thigh   With the lower hand on the back of the knee for support, reach across the athlete and use your fingers to locate the groove that runs next to the hamstrings. That is the iliotibial band. Administer local cross-fiber strokes the length of the band, from the buttock almost to the knee. These strokes should last approximately ten seconds. Cover the length of the band at least twice.

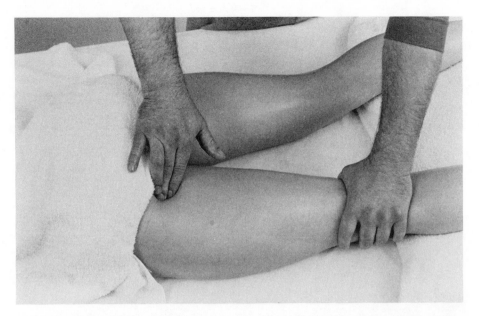

Local Cross-Fiber Stroking at the Origin of the Hamstring Reach across the table and stabilize the knee of the far leg with your lower hand. With the fingers of your upper hand, find the origin of the hamstring just below the buttock. Apply local cross-fiber strokes for at least three minutes, using as much pressure as possible.

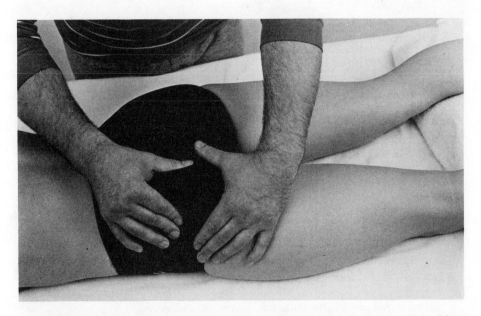

Kneading the Buttock From next to the hip, reach across the athlete and knead the buttock with the thumb and fingers from the cheek almost to the lower back. Cover the area up and down three times.

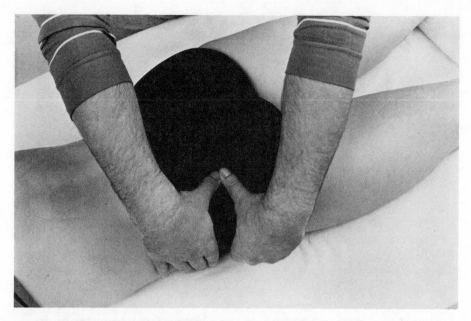

Broad Cross-Fiber Stroking of the Buttock   Reach across the athlete with both hands and administer broad cross-fiber strokes across the entire buttock with your thumbs, pulling across the muscle to the hip. Cover it at least twice with strokes.

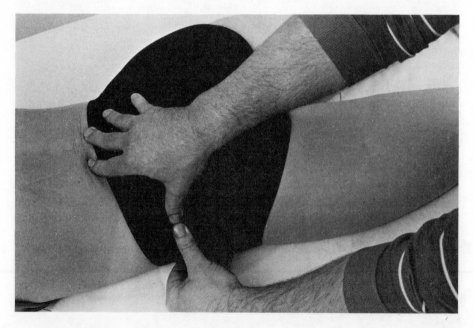

Deep Stroking of the Buttock   From a position next to the leg you are massaging, deep-stroke the buttock, putting your thumbs tip to tip and stroking up the buttock in rows. Cover the entire buttock from cheek to lower back at least twice.

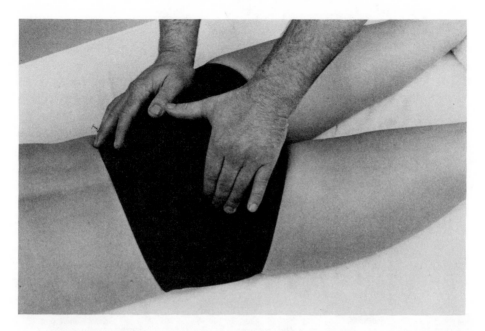

Local Cross-Fiber Stroking of the Buttock Reach across the athlete and locate the rim of the buttock with the tips of the middle and forefingers. It is just above the hip. Apply local cross-fiber strokes to this rim, lifting the muscle away from the bone. Each of the local cross-fiber strokes should last about ten seconds. Cover this area at least twice. Repeat on the other side.

Back Warm-up

Before performing the curative strokes on the back, perform the following warm-up movements.

Light Stroking with Two Hands With hands placed fingertip to fingertip over the spine, stroke up to the midback, covering about one foot per movement. Cover this area about three times.

Kneading the Lower Back From a position next to the athlete's waist, reach across and knead the lower back. Cover the area at least three times before moving to the other side of the athlete and performing these movements on the other side of the back.

Fanning of the Lower Back From a position next to the athlete's buttocks, fan the lower back, placing the hands in prayer fashion on the spine and pushing down and spreading out the hands. Repeat at least three times and begin the curative routine.

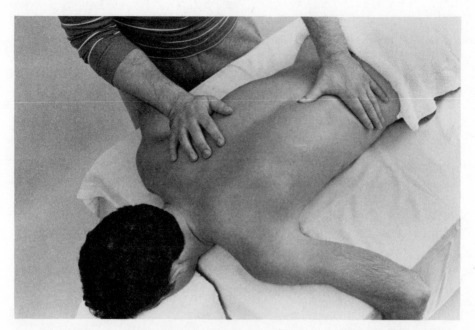

Broad Cross-Fiber Stroking of the Muscles of the Spine (Spinal Erec-tors) From next to the athlete's chest, place your upper hand between the shoulders and administer broad cross-fiber strokes to the muscles along the outside portion of the spine. Push across these muscles with your thumb from the lower back to the middle of the back. Repeat three times. Switch sides and perform the same movements on the other side of the spine.

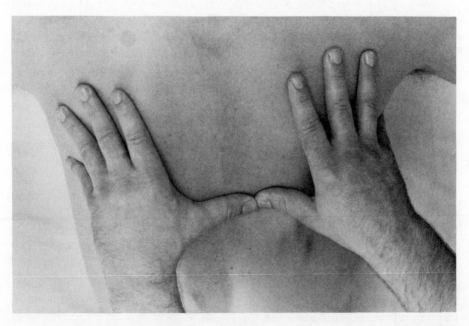

Deep Stroking of the Muscles of the Spine From a position next to the athlete's waist, bring the thumbs together over the muscles on one side of the spine. Deep-stroke from the lower back to the base of the shoulder blades in one smooth, continuous movement. Cover one side of the spine three times, then repeat on the other side of the spine.

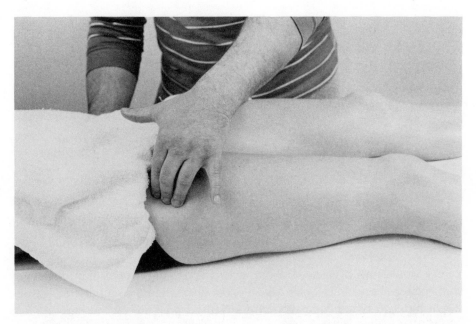

Local Cross-Fiber Stroking of the Hip Muscle (Tensor Fascia Lata) Have the athlete turn over onto his back. Reaching across the body, find the tensor fascia latae, which is located at the top and to the outside of the quadriceps, where these muscles join the hip. Administer local cross-fiber strokes that last approximately ten seconds. Repeat at least three times on each side.

16 · SHINS

Shin splints are most common to the young athlete and the new athlete, but they can happen to an athlete at any level. Just ask Mary Decker.

For years, Mary was afflicted by shin splints so severe that she thought her career would end because of them. It was finally discovered that the sheath that encloses her shin muscles wasn't expanding when the muscles did, resulting in reduced blood circulation and increased pressure on the nerves. As a result, surgery has twice been performed on Mary's shins to split the sheath and allow the muscles to expand freely.

Fortunately, most shin splints can be corrected nonsurgically. They are usually caused by fatigue of the lower leg muscles where the tendons attach to the front and/or rear of the tibia, the weight-bearing shinbone.

Exercising gradually strengthens these muscles and tendons. But too much exercise can irritate them. Unfortunately, we rarely know what too much exercise is until after we feel its effects.

This massage will relieve the calf tension that is sometimes responsible for shin tightness. It also improves circulation to the shins and relieves tightness in the tendons at the top and bottom of the shins.

Shin splints are unmistakable—if you have them, your shins feel sore when you walk, on fire when you run.

In addition to the curative massage (which should be performed once a day) there are some other things you should do to deal with shin splints. Ice helps. Applied twice a day for twenty minutes per shin, it will increase blood flow to the afflicted area. Strengthening the shin muscles will also help. Lifting a weight with the lower leg (for example, lifting a bucket of water or sand with the toes by picking up and straightening the lower leg while sitting) will increase the strength of this area. A softer running surface (if you are a runner) or shoes with better cushioning will also help, since shin splints are frequently caused by impact.

Warm-up

Before administering the curative strokes for the shins, perform the following warm-up routine.

Light Stroking of the Shin   From a position by the athlete's foot, begin at the ankle and light-stroke the shin with the palms of the hands. Continue the stroke until just before the knee and then glide the palms back down to the ankle. Repeat this movement at least three times.

Kneading of the Shin   From a position next to the shin, reach across the athlete and knead the outside portion of the shin of the far leg. Knead from the ankle to just below the knee and back again. Repeat this movement three times, then begin the curative routine.

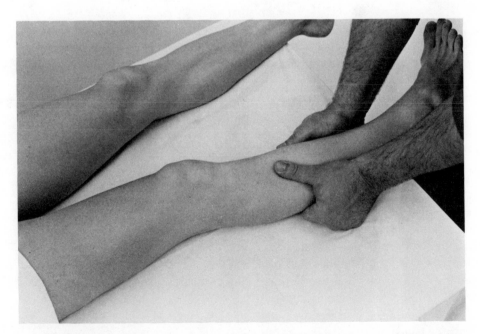

Broad Cross-Fiber Stroking of the Shin   Positioning yourself beneath the athlete's feet, hold the inside of the calf with your inside hand. With the thumb of the outside hand, cover the outside of the shin with broad cross-fiber strokes from just above the ankle to just below the knee. Repeat three times.

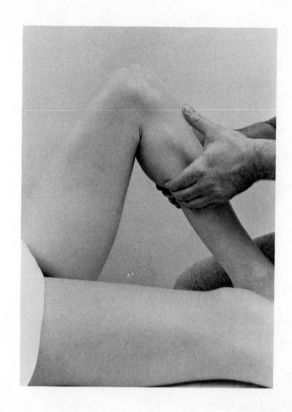

Deep Stroking of the Shins With the athlete's knee up and the foot resting on the table, put your fingers around the calf and deep-stroke the shins toward the knee with your thumbs. Cover the area as hard as possible, remembering that this is a tender area. Repeat at least three times.

Local Cross-Fiber Stroking of the Top of the Foot With your lower hand holding the bottom of the foot, locate the tendons on the outside top of the athlete's foot. Administer local cross-fiber strokes with the tips of the fingers, probing the tendons across the top of the foot. Cover this area at least three times.

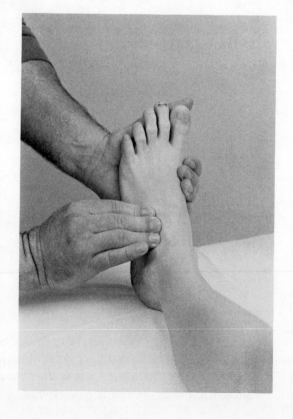

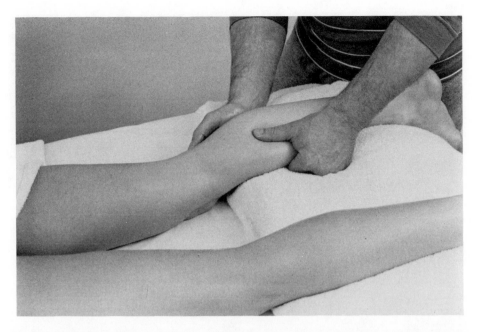

Broad Cross-Fiber Stroking of the Calf With the athlete on his stomach, stabilize the outside of the leg with your outside hand held against the
knee. With the thumb of the inside hand, administer broad cross-fiber strokes
to the calf, moving in rows from above the Achilles tendon to just below the
knee. Cover the calf three times.

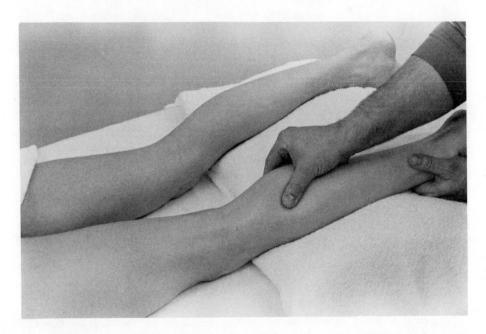

Jostling of the Calf Holding the ankle with your outside hand, grasp
the calf with the thumb and fingers of your inside hand and jostle the muscle
vigorously for about thirty seconds. Repeat three times.

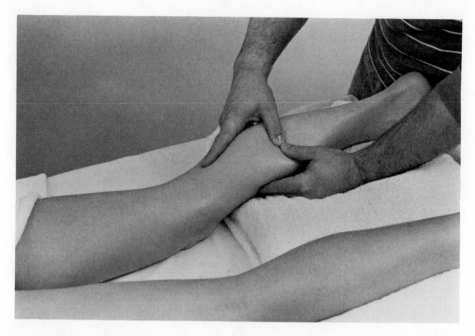

Deep Stroking of the Calf   Placing your fingers on either side of the calf, bring the thumbs together and stroke up the calf, from the top of the Achilles to just below the knee. Cover the entire calf three times.

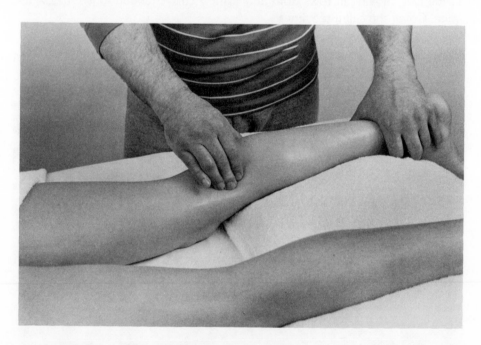

Local Cross-Fiber Stroking of the Tendons at the Top of the Calf
From a position next to the athlete's knee, find the top of the calf muscle where it attaches to the back of the knee. With your fingertips, cross the attachment several times, each lasting at least ten seconds. Repeat at least three times.

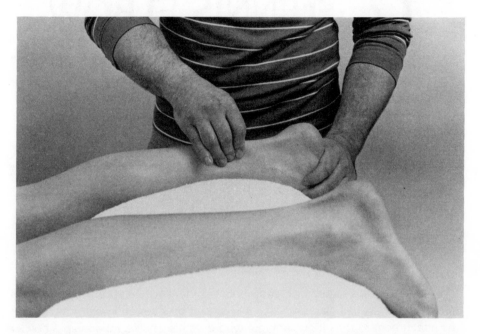

Local Cross-Fiber Stroking of the Base of the Calf With your finger-tips, find the base of the calf. Apply local cross-fiber strokes to the area for at least ten seconds. Repeat at least three times.

17 · TENNIS ELBOW

Elbow injury is the scourge of tennis and all other racquet sports; it sometimes affects even baseball players. Since it is caused by strained forearm muscles at the attachment to the elbow, anyone who uses his wrists a lot—even a bowler —is susceptible to this injury.

The cause of tennis elbow can range from a racquet or balls that are too heavy to improper stroking or using the wrist instead of the entire arm to make shots.

But some causes can't be remedied. Muscles by their very nature shorten when they are used. And when the forearm muscles shorten they put undue strain on the tendons at the elbow.

Tennis elbow is different from simple soreness of the elbow. For one thing, it doesn't go away after a few minutes of play as ordinary soreness does. The elbow is frequently sore to the touch, especially around the knobs at the joint. And it hurts at the elbow when the forearm is flexed.

If these symptoms are present, rest the area, apply ice for no more than ten minutes twice daily and follow the curative massage routine below once a day. Do not massage the elbow for the first twenty-four to forty-eight hours after the injury.

The curative strokes outlined here include massage of the upper arm as well as the forearm. The shortening of any arm muscles causes stress at the elbow, which is why they are treated. In addition to preventing muscle shortening, massage will bring blood to the area of the tendons to aid in healing.

Warm-up

Before beginning the curative strokes, perform the following warm-up routine.

Light Stroking of the Arm   With the athlete's arm flat on the table, place the palms of your hands on top of each other (for controlled pressure) and stroke gently up the arm to the top of the shoulder. Slide your palms back down the arm and repeat the procedure, this time more firmly. Repeat a third time, still more firmly. Then turn the palm up and repeat the strokes.

Kneading of the Arm   Using the thumbs and fingers of both hands, knead the arm from the wrist to the biceps, including parts of the shoulder, and then back down again. After the arm has been kneaded up and down three times, begin the curative routine.

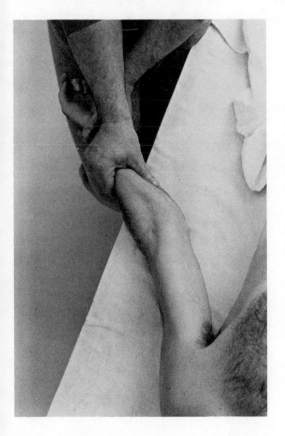

Broad Cross-Fiber Stroking of the Inside of the Forearm   Holding the athlete's wrist so the palm is up, cover the arm from the wrist to the elbow with broad cross-fiber strokes. Begin gently, increasing the pressure with each subsequent pass. If the athlete tenses the area, ease the pressure of the strokes. Cover the area at least four times.

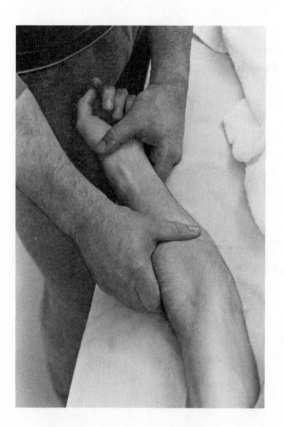

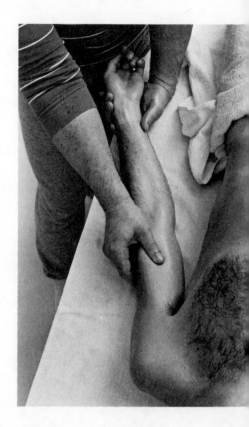

Deep Stroking of the Forearm Still holding the athlete's wrist with your lower hand, administer deep strokes to the inside of the forearm with the thumb of your upper hand. Cover the entire forearm three times from the wrist to just below the biceps.

Broad Cross-Fiber Stroking of the Biceps Still holding the athlete's wrist with your lower hand, cross the biceps with the thumb of your upper hand in rows from the top to the bottom and back again. Repeat three times.

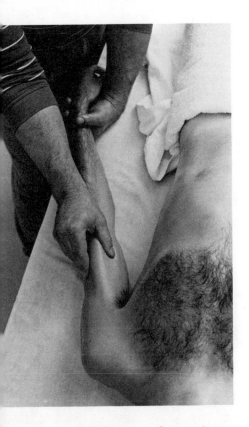

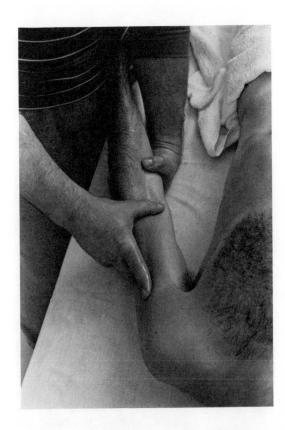

Jostling of the Biceps Grasp the athlete's biceps between your thumb and fingers and jostle vigorously for about thirty seconds. Repeat this movement three times.

Deep Stroking of the Biceps Holding the athlete's forearm with your lower hand, administer deep strokes the length of the biceps, from just above the elbow almost to the shoulder. Cover the entire biceps at least three times.

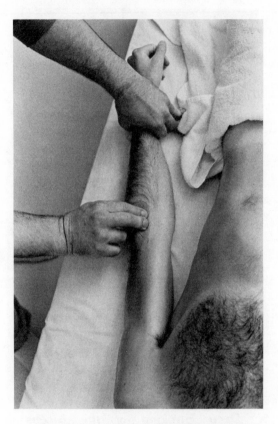

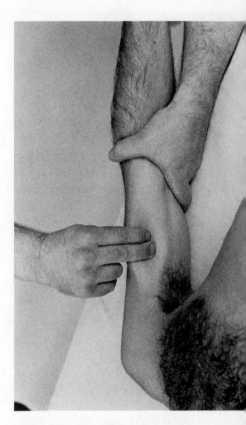

Local Cross-Fiber Stroking of the Tendons Below the Elbow Wipe the oil from the skin. Holding the athlete's wrist to the table with your lower hand, use the upper hand to administer local cross-fiber strokes to the tendons just below the elbow. Cross the tendons with the tips of your forefinger and middle finger for as long as two minutes, pressing progressively harder.

Local Cross-Fiber Stroking of the Biceps (Optional: use when muscles feel tight or when knots are felt) Holding the athlete's elbow with your lower hand, administer local cross-fiber strokes to the biceps with the forefinger and middle finger of your upper hand. Cross the biceps in finger-wide rows. Cover the biceps at least three times.

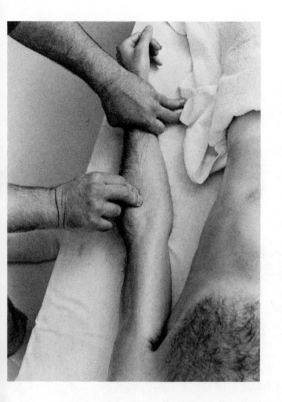

***Local Cross-Fiber Stroking of the
Biceps Insertion*** Remove oil from
the elbow area with a towel. Holding
the athlete's arm stable with your
lower hand, use the fingertips of the
upper hand to isolate the tendons that
join at the elbow from the upper and
lower arm. They feel like strings beneath the skin. Apply cross-fiber
strokes to these tendons with your fingertips. Your goal is to loosen these
tight tendons, but make sure it isn't a
painful experience for the athlete.
Stroke the area for two to three minutes.

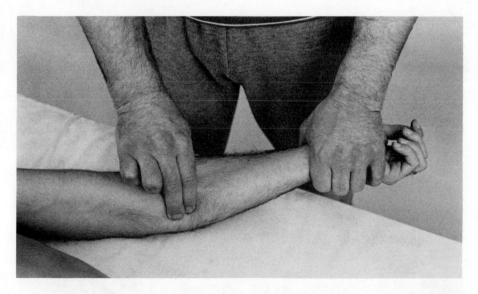

Local Cross-Fiber Stroking of the Forearm Insertion With the athlete
on his back, grasp the wrist with the lower hand for stability. With the upper
hand, locate the tendons of the forearm with the tips of your middle and
forefinger. When you find them (they, too, will feel like strings under the skin),
execute local cross-fiber strokes across them with the tips of your fingers for
two to three minutes.

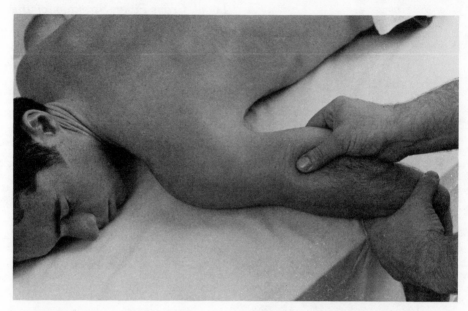

Broad Cross-Fiber Stroking of the Triceps With the athlete on his stomach, hold the elbow with the upper hand and administer broad cross-fiber strokes to the triceps, moving from the elbow almost to the shoulder. Cover the area three times.

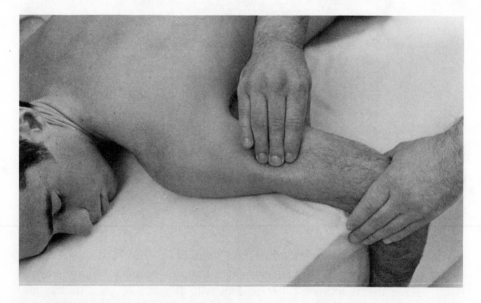

Jostling of the Triceps With the upper hand holding the athlete's elbow, jostle the triceps with the lower hand for about a minute. This will loosen the muscles in preparation for deep stroking.

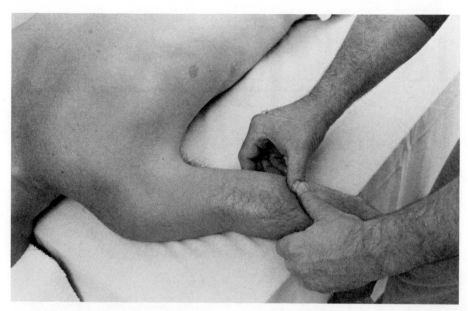

Deep Stroking of the Triceps With the fingers on either side of the upper arm for stability, bring your thumbs together (one on top of the other, if you need the additional strength) and deep-stroke the triceps from the elbow to the shoulder. Repeat at least three times.

18 · UPPER LEGS
(Hamstrings, Groin, and Knees)

Grab the back of your upper leg. That is the hamstring muscle, which runs from the bottom of the pelvis to the back of the knee. And if you suddenly grab it in pain while exercising, chances are good that you have a strained hamstring.

It's easy to diagnose. For one thing, you feel an acute soreness in the muscle. The pain increases from the point where you first felt it, and sometimes you may feel swelling with your fingertips. In cases of severe swelling, a black-and-blue mark may actually be seen.

Groin injuries are different. Because of the chunkiness of this muscle, which is near the crotch where it pulls the legs together, strains don't manifest themselves as quickly as they do in the thinner muscles. They come on more slowly and frequently, become chronic (meaning they are strained longer than six weeks), because the athlete doesn't notice them as soon and continues to work out through what he thinks is ordinary muscle soreness.

Knee problems vary a great deal. I have seen them occur quickly and I have seen them develop over a period of several days—sometimes several weeks.

The knee consists primarily of tendons and ligaments. It suffers injury not only from strains to the joint itself, but also from shortening of the muscles of the upper and lower leg with tendon attachments at the knee. Based on my experience, the knee is more susceptible to injury than even the Achilles tendon.

On the first sign of injury to any of these areas, stop exercising, or at least cut down. Apply ice to the afflicted area at least twice per day, ten minutes per session. And apply curative massage once a day to the injured area of the leg.

This massage will loosen and spread fibers in the main body of the hamstring and will improve circulation throughout the muscle and the tendons coming from the muscles.

Warm-up

Before beginning the curative strokes for the hamstrings, perform the following warm-up routine.

Light Stroking of the Hamstring With the athlete lying face down, assume a position next to the knee and stroke gently with the palms of your hands, from the back of the knee to the buttock. Glide the palms back. Repeat the movement at least three times.

Kneading of the Back of the Leg From a position next to the athlete's upper leg, begin kneading the inside of the upper leg from the knee to the buttock and back. Repeat at least three times, making sure to cover the entire back of the upper leg. Begin the curative routine.

Hamstrings

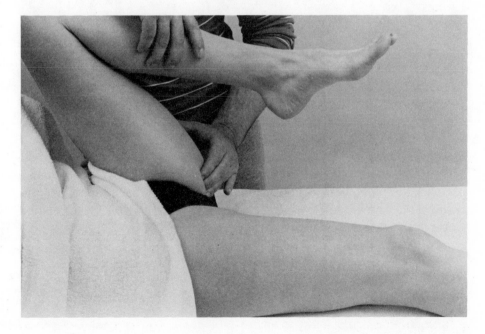

Local Cross-Fiber Stroking of the Hamstring with the Knee Up From next to the athlete's hip, hold the shin of the leg closest to you with your upper hand and bring the knee up and the foot off the table as shown. With your fingers, find the origin of the hamstring, which is at the base of the buttock. Cross back and forth over the origin of the hamstring for at least a minute, applying progressively more pressure.

This position is used because the origin of the hamstring is sometimes difficult to find and control when the athlete is lying on his stomach.

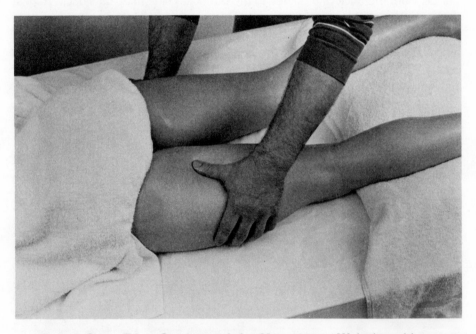

Broad Cross-Fiber Stroking of the Hamstring With the athlete now lying on his stomach, stroke across the hamstring of the far leg with the thumb of your lower hand, from just above the knee to the point of insertion near the cheek of the buttock. Apply as much pressure as is comfortable for the athlete. Cover this muscle at least three times.

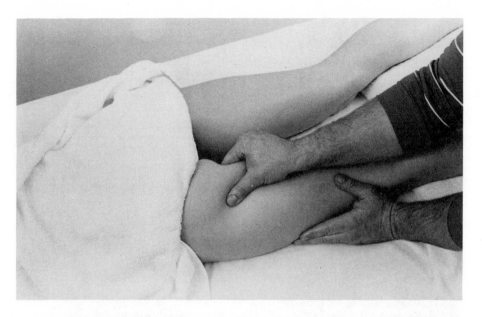

Jostling of the Hamstring From next to the athlete's knee, stabilize the leg with your upper hand and grasp the hamstring with your lower hand. Jostle the muscle vigorously for at least thirty seconds. Repeat three times.

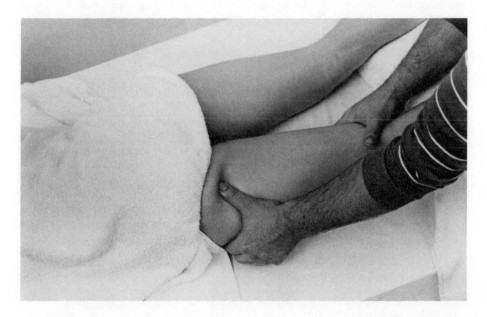

Deep Stroking of the Hamstring With one hand on the inside portion of the knee closest to you, stroke the athlete's hamstring lengthwise with your thumb. The stroke, which begins just above the knee and continues to the cheek of the buttock, should be as deep as the athlete can tolerate. Repeat at least three times. If you need more pressure, use both thumbs, one on top of the other.

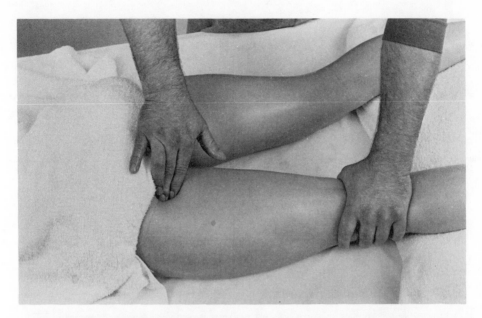

Local Cross-Fiber Stroking Near the Origin of the Hamstring With the tips of your middle and forefinger, locate the origin of the hamstring, which is just below the cheek of the buttock. Administer local cross-fiber strokes to this area, tenderly at first and then applying more pressure. Since small tears are frequent here and may have left deposits of scar tissue, this may be a sore area. Local cross-fiber strokes should last about ten seconds. Perform at least four of them.

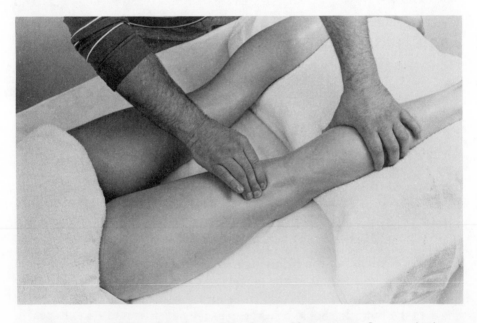

Local Cross-Fiber Stroking of the Lower Hamstring Locate the lower portion of the hamstring with your fingertips; it is just above the back of the knee. Holding the leg stable with your lower hand, administer local cross-fiber strokes with your fingertips to any tense areas. These are likely to be sore, so probe gently. Local cross-fiber strokes should last about ten seconds. Repeat at least three times over each area of tension.

Groin

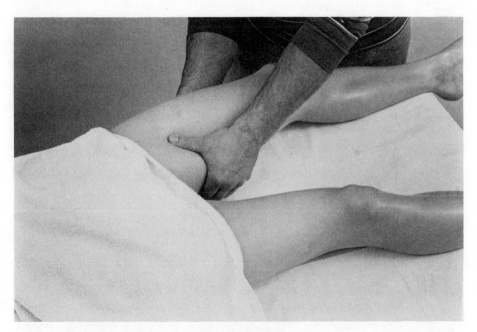

Broad Cross-Fiber Stroking of the Groin With the athlete on his back, stand next to his knee. Stabilizing the outside of the thigh with your upper hand, wrap the fingers of your lower hand around the groin and apply broad cross-fiber strokes with the thumb, covering the groin in rows up to the crotch. Repeat three times.

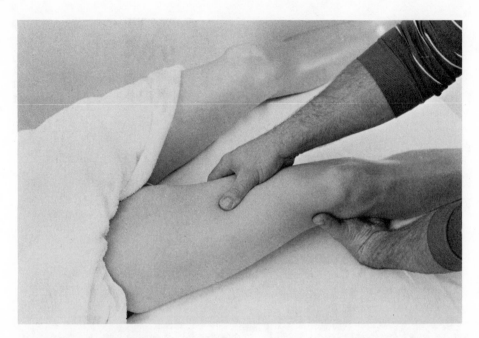

Jostling of the Groin Stabilizing the athlete's leg with the upper hand, grasp the groin with the lower hand and jostle the muscle for at least thirty seconds. Repeat three times.

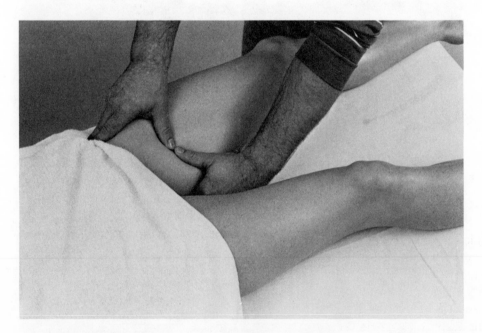

Deep Stroking of the Top of the Thigh (Adductors) Straddle the athlete's thigh with your hands, bringing your thumbs together to apply deep strokes to the front of the thigh. Cover the area three times.

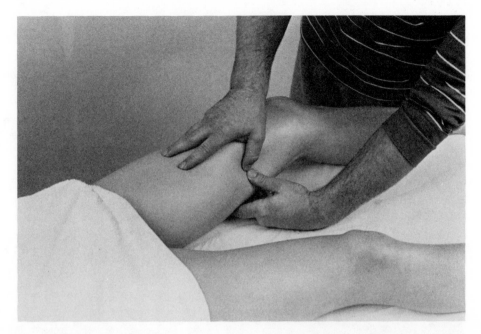

Deep Stroking of the Inside of the Leg (Gracilis) Place your thumbs on the inside portion of the upper leg and stroke up in rows, almost to the crotch. Apply moderate pressure at first, stroking deeper with each pass. Cover the entire area at least three times.

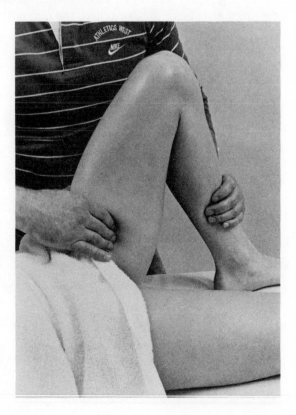

Local Cross-Fiber Stroking of the Top of the Thigh (Adductors) With the athlete's knee up and your hand just above the ankle for support, apply local cross-fiber strokes to any area of tension felt in that area. Cover each area as deeply as possible at least three times.

This massage is to spread and loosen the fibers of the groin and improve circulation to the area.

Thighs and Knees

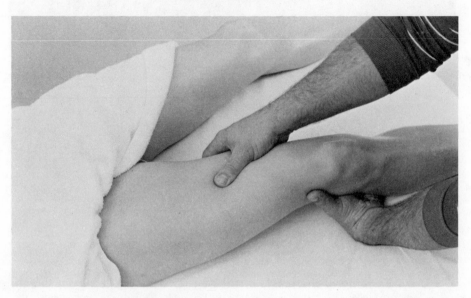

Broad Cross-Fiber Stroking of the Quadriceps From next to the athlete's feet and with your upper hand holding the knee of the leg closest to you for stability, apply broad cross-fiber strokes to the quadriceps. Stroke the muscles from just above the knee up to the groin. Repeat at least three times.

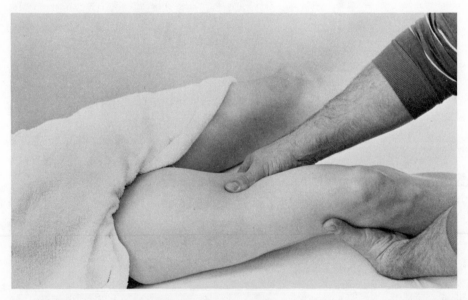

Jostling of the Quadriceps From next to the athlete's shins, stabilize the outside of the knee with your upper hand. With the lower hand, grasp the quadriceps and jostle them vigorously for at least thirty seconds. Repeat three times.

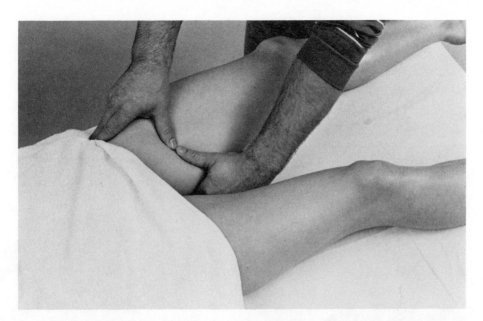

Deep Stroking of the Quadriceps From next to the athlete's knee, place your fingers on either side of the athlete's thigh. Bring your thumbs together and deep-stroke the quadriceps in rows almost to the crotch. Repeat three times.

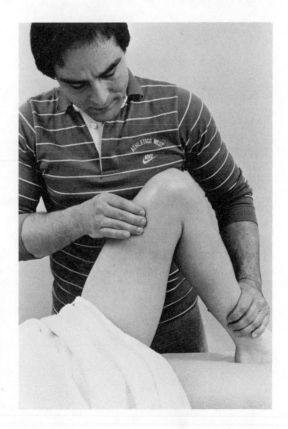

Local Cross-Fiber Stroking of Knots in Quadriceps (optional) If you locate a knot in the vastus medialis or other portions of the quadriceps, raise the knee and treat the knot with local cross-fiber strokes. Cross the knot several times, applying increased pressure to the area. Repeat at least four times.

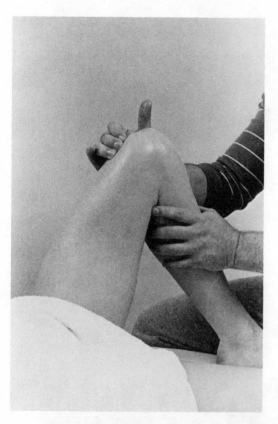

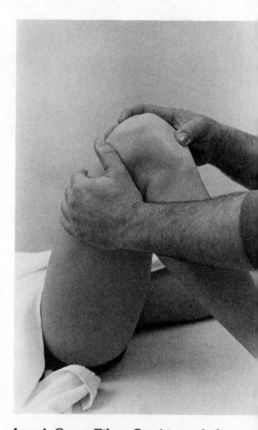

***Local Cross-Fiber Stroking of the
Patella Tendon Above the Knee***
With the knee raised, find the tendon above the kneecap with your fingertips. Administer local cross-fiber strokes of approximately ten seconds in duration, increasing the pressure with subsequent strokes. Repeat at least three times.

***Local Cross-Fiber Stroking of the
Patella Tendon Below the Knee***
With the knee still raised, locate the tendon below the kneecap. Administer several local cross-fiber movements of about ten seconds' duration. Repeat at least three times.

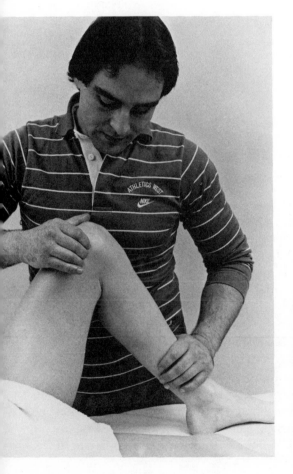

Local Cross-Fiber Stroking of the Muscle Inside the Knee (Sartorius) With the knee still elevated, place your fingertips near the knee joint on the inside of the leg closest to you. Apply local cross-fiber strokes to the area as deeply as the athlete can tolerate. Cover the area at least three times with strokes lasting approximately ten seconds.

19 · SHOULDERS

Given the versatility of the shoulders it is no wonder they are an area of frequent injury. Baseball, football and racquet sports all tax the tendons and muscles of the shoulders. Even swimming, a seemingly gentle sport, tests the shoulder's unique ability to rotate 360 degrees.

The framework for the shoulder is formed by a girdle of bones to which the large skeletal muscles attach. These muscles come from the chest, the back and the base of the neck. They provide the structural stability of the shoulder as well as much of the power it delivers.

Around those large muscles are several smaller ones that perform such duties as holding the ball joint of the arm tightly against the shoulder socket. And tying all of this together like so much twine are many ligaments and tendons all of which are areas of potential stress.

Diagnosing a shoulder strain is easy: it hurts. Sometimes it hurts only when you execute a certain movement, such as lateral raises with dumbbells, for instance. Other times—if it is worse—it hurts whenever any stress is placed upon it.

The best treatment for an injured shoulder is rest. Without that, curative massage will have little long-term effect. Ice will also help the afflicted area by improving the blood's circulation and reducing edema to speed healing. Ice treatments should take place twice a day, twenty minutes per session. Rest and ice should be supplements to the following curative massage routine.

Warm-up

Before beginning the curative strokes, prepare the muscles with the following warm-up routine.

Light Stroking of the Upper Back From a position next to the athlete's back, place the hands fingertip to fingertip over the spine and rub up to the shoulders from the middle of the back. Glide the palms back down and repeat the movement at least three times.

Light Stroking of the Chest With the athlete on his back, stand next to the chest and place the palms of your hands on the bottom of the rib cage beneath the sternum. Administer light strokes out to the front of the deltoids. Repeat, covering the entire chest at least three times.

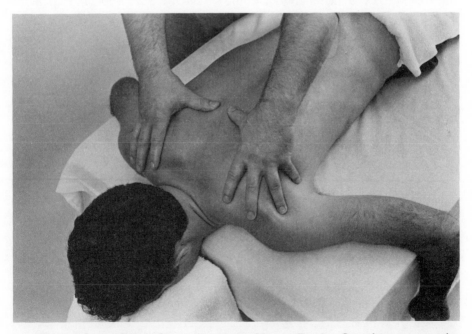

Broad Cross-Fiber Stroking of the Upper Back Standing next to the athlete's waist, put a hand on each shoulder blade. Put the thumbs on either side of the spine and stroke up to the base of the trapezius. Cover the area between the shoulder blades and spine three times.

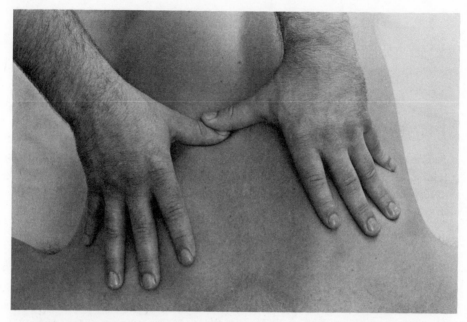

Deep Stroking of the Upper Back Placing your thumbs on one side of the spine, administer deep strokes from the midback almost to the neck. Cover the area in rows to the inner edge of the shoulder blade (scapula). Repeat this massage at least three times.

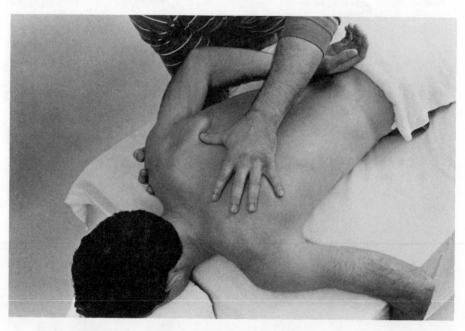

Broad Cross-Fiber Stroking of the Upper Back with Elevated Shoulder Blade (Scapula) Place the top of the athlete's hand closest to you on his lower back, as shown. This causes the shoulder blade to become prominent, with easy-to-follow contours. Administer broad cross-fiber strokes to the area between the shoulder blade and the spine, stroking parallel to the spine with the thumb of the lower hand and as deep as possible, to effectively massage these thick muscles. Cover the area at least three times.

Then return the arm to its resting position on the table and administer broad cross-fiber strokes over the shoulder blade with the thumb of the lower hand. Move up in rows, from the bottom of the shoulder blade to the top. Cover the area three times.

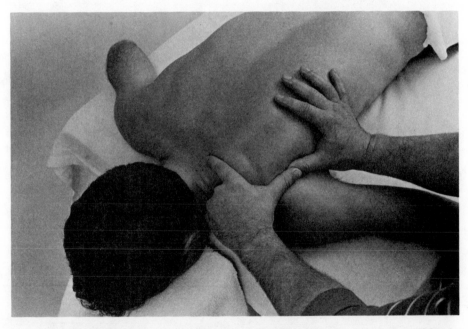

Deep Stroking Over the Shoulder Blade From next to the athlete's shoulder, place your thumbs together and administer deep strokes from the shoulder joint to the midback. Cross the shoulder blade in rows. Cover it three times.

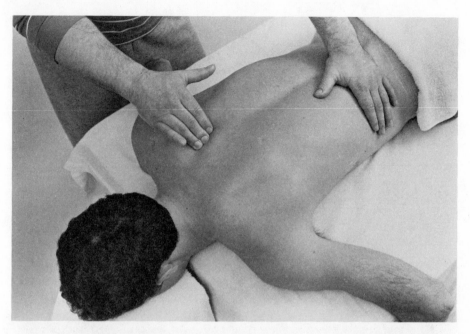

Local Cross-Fiber Stroking of the Muscles Along the Spine (Spinal Erectors) With the fingertips of your upper hand, locate the muscles next to the spine on the side of the athlete's spine closest to you. Administer local cross-fiber strokes to the muscles, stroking back and forth from the midline out (not parallel to the spine). Cover the muscles up to the shoulder blade. Repeat at least three times.

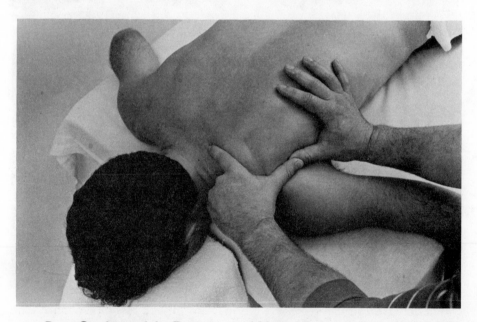

Deep Stroking of the Posterior and Medial Deltoid With both thumbs on the athlete's deltoid, stroke toward the head in rows, covering the area as deeply as possible. Repeat at least three times.

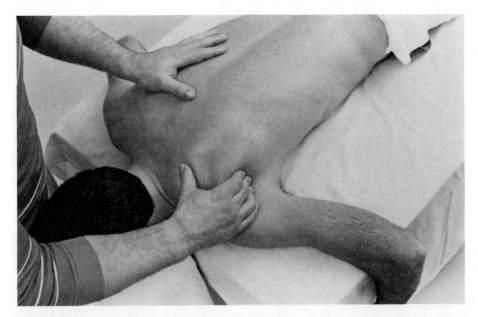

Local Cross-Fiber Stroking of the Muscles Around the Shoulder Blade (Teres Minor, Infraspinatus and Teres Major) Locate these muscles, which are just above the armpit and in from the deltoid. With your fingertips, administer local cross-fiber strokes to any areas of tension felt during the massage of the shoulder blade. A minute or two will loosen the tension noticeably. Cover these muscles as deeply as comfort permits, at least three times.

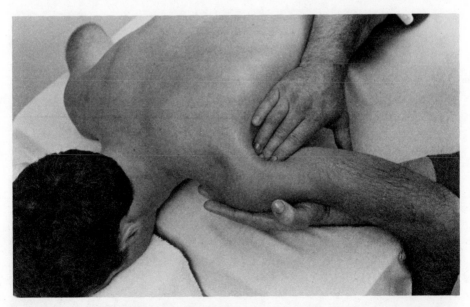

Local Cross-Fiber Stroking of the Posterior and Medial Deltoid With the palm of the upper hand beneath the deltoid, administer local cross-fiber strokes to the posterior portion, moving back and forth with the fingertips as deeply as possible, applying additional pressure to knots.

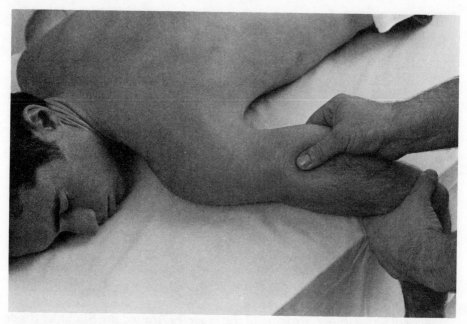

Broad Cross-Fiber Stroking of the Triceps   Holding the athlete's elbow with your upper hand, stroke across the triceps with the thumb of your lower hand in rows from just above the elbow to the deltoid. Repeat three times.

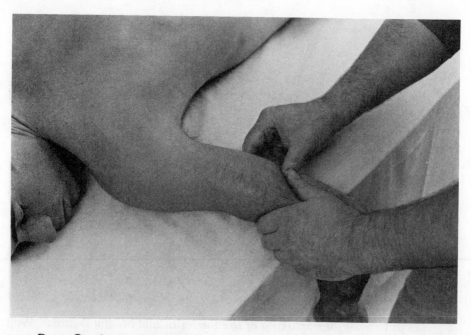

Deep Stroking of the Triceps   Placing your thumbs together over the triceps, deep-stroke in rows from the elbow to the deltoid. Cover the muscle with strokes. Repeat three times.

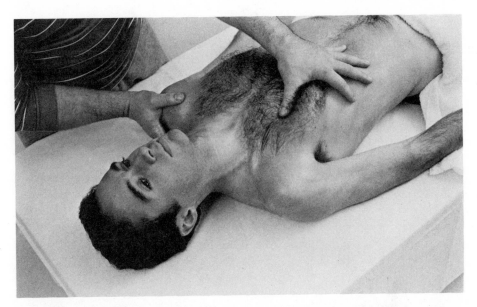

Broad Cross-Fiber Stroking of the Chest (Pectoralis Major) Have the athlete lie on his back. From next to his waist, reach across to the opposite side of the chest and administer broad cross-fiber strokes from the middle of the chest to the deltoid. Cover the area in rows. Repeat three times.

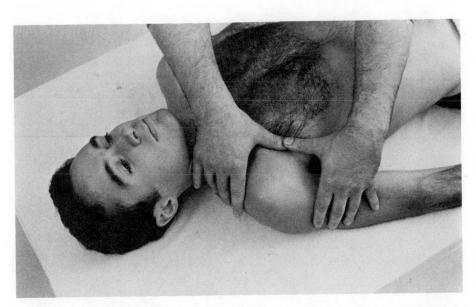

Deep Stroking of the Pectoralis Major With the athlete on his back, locate the pectoralis on the side farthest from you. With the pad of your thumb, deep-stroke from the sternum toward the shoulder. Cover the entire area up to the collarbone as deeply as possible, applying as much pressure as the athlete is comfortable with. Repeat at least three times.

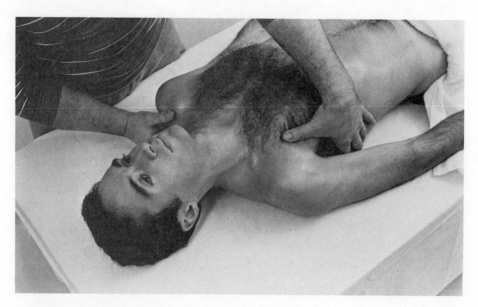

Deep Stroking the Front of the Deltoid From next to the athlete's shoulder, reach across with your lower hand and apply deep strokes to the front of the deltoid. Stroke in rows out to the end of the shoulder. Cover the entire front of the deltoid three times.

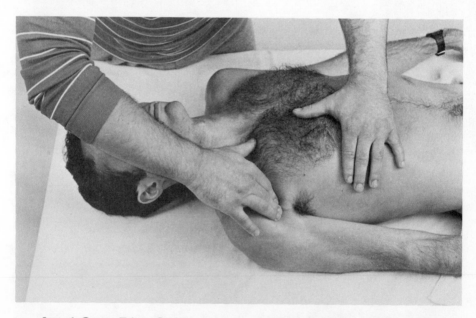

Local Cross-Fiber Stroking of the Frontal Deltoid With your lower hand on the opposite side of the athlete's chest for support, locate the deltoid with the fingertips of your other hand. Apply local cross-fiber strokes parallel to the body and in rows moving toward you. Cover any tense areas of the deltoid at least three times.

Broad Cross-Fiber Stroking of the Biceps From next to the athlete's waist, hold the nearby wrist with your lower hand and administer broad cross-fiber strokes to the biceps with your upper hand, moving in rows from just above the elbow to the deltoid. Repeat three times.

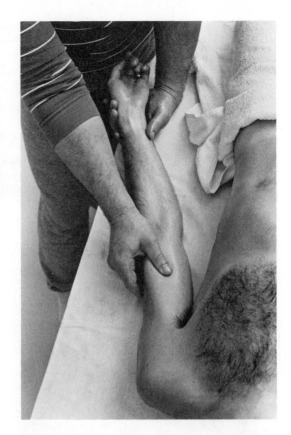

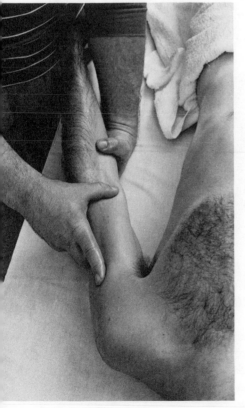

Deep Stroking of the Biceps Holding the elbow with your lower hand, deep-stroke the biceps with the thumb of your upper hand, covering it in rows from the elbow to the armpit. Repeat three times.

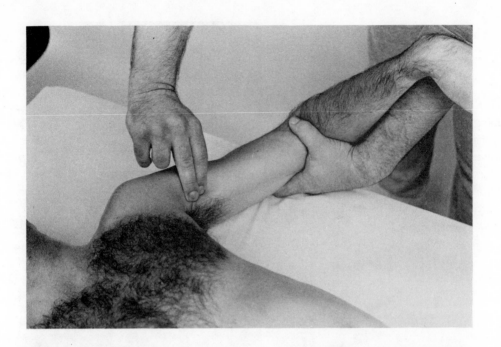

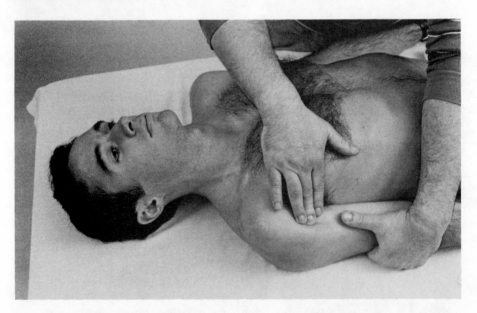

***Local Cross-Fiber Stroking of the Biceps' Two Tendon
Attachments*** Holding the athlete's arm with your lower hand, pull the elbow
away from the body. With the middle and forefingers of your upper hand,
administer local cross-fiber strokes to the inside tendon attachment of the
biceps near the armpit. Apply strokes for about ten seconds. Release pressure.
Repeat three times.

Moving the athlete's elbow back to his side, locate the biceps tendon just
beneath the deltoid. Administer local cross-fiber strokes for at least ten seconds.
Release pressure. Repeat three times.

20 · NECK

The neck contains the cervical spine, the most vulnerable portion of the spinal cord, which carries messages from the brain to all portions of the body.

For many athletes, the neck and trapezius represent a great source of stress, for others, just a plain old headache. Many athletes carry a lot of stress in their neck and shoulders. Some do so because they hunch their shoulders in training or athletic competition. Others suffer from spasms to their neck muscles because the muscles aren't strong enough to sustain activity, and so they spasm to prevent real injury to the area.

Whatever the causes—and there are many potential ones—it is these spasms that put pressure on nerves and cause pain and stiffness in the neck and shoulder regions. And it is these neck spasms that curative massage can most effectively treat.

Because of the contour of the neck and the bony configuration of the spine, massage to this area can be somewhat painful. Begin the massage gently, even if pressed for time. Discomfort to the area will be counterproductive to the relaxation effort.

Neck pain that is accompanied by pain down the arms is a condition that should be examined by an orthopedic doctor. Such symptoms could point to disc damage, which is a problem that massage won't remedy.

The first nine photos in this chapter show Alberto Salazar lying face down into side-by-side cushions which are a special attachment to my massage table. You can approximate this position by placing a thick pillow under the athlete's chest and having him rest his forehead on the floor. If there is no table for the athlete to drape his arms from, place the arms back by the athlete's sides.

Warm-up

Light Stroking of the Neck   With the athlete on his stomach, arms to his sides, stroke firmly with the fingertips from the base of the skull to the shoulders. Thoroughly cover the neck and trapezius at least three times.

Petrissage of the Neck and Shoulders   To further loosen the muscles of the neck and shoulders, stand at the head of the table and administer circular strokes from the base of the skull to the end of the trapezius. Repeat at least three times.

Kneading of the Trapezius   From next to the athlete, grasp the trapezius between the thumbs and fingers of both hands, kneading on either side of the neck and moving out toward the ends of the muscle. Repeat three times. Begin the curative routine.

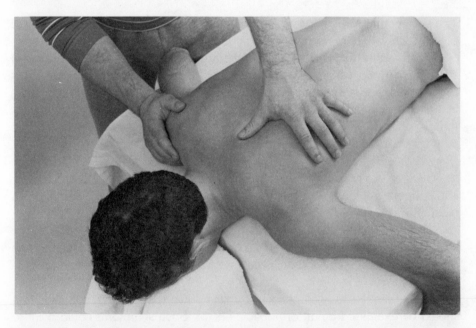

Broad Cross-Fiber Stroking at the Muscles Along the Spine (Spinal Erectors)   From next to the athlete's shoulder, use the thumb of the lower hand to administer broad cross-fiber strokes to the muscles on the opposite side of the spine. Cover the area from midback to the base of the neck with strokes at least three times. Change sides and repeat the procedure on the other side of the spine.

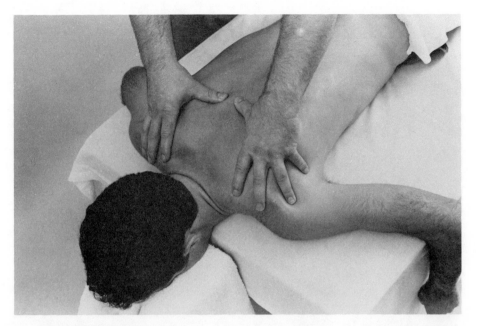

Deep Stroking of the Muscles Along the Spine From next to the athlete's waist, place your thumbs on each side of the spine and administer deep strokes to the muscles of the spine, stroking from the middle of the back to the base of the neck. Cover the area slowly and deeply at least three times.

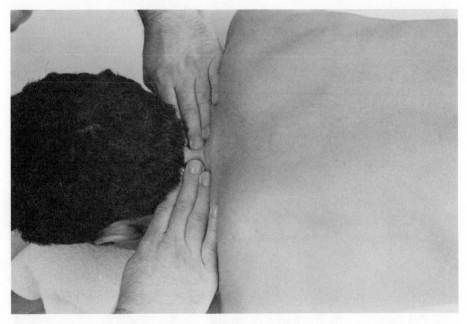

Light Stroking of the Neck From above the athlete's head, light-stroke his neck with your fingertips, moving up and down the neck at least four times.

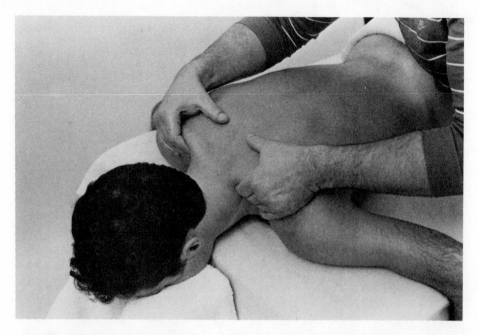

Kneading of the Trapezius From next to the athlete, place your hands on either side of the neck and knead the trapezius with your thumbs and fingers. Knead the length of the muscle from the base of the neck out to the end and back. Cover the area at least three times.

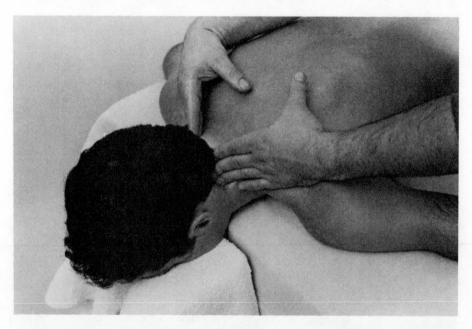

Petrissage of the Neck and Trapezius Using your fingertips, administer petrissage from the base of the skull to the ends of the trapezius and back, applying progressively deeper strokes. Cover the area at least three times.

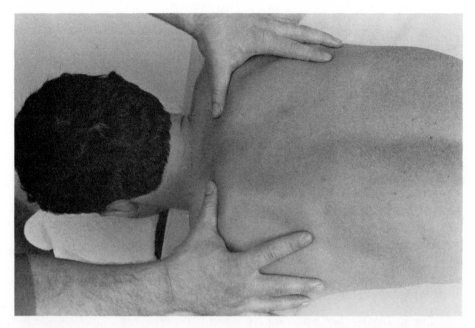

Broad Cross-Fiber Stroking of the Trapezius Placing the thumbs on either side of the athlete's neck, push straight down, ending the stroke at the shoulder blades. Cover the upper back in rows at least three times.

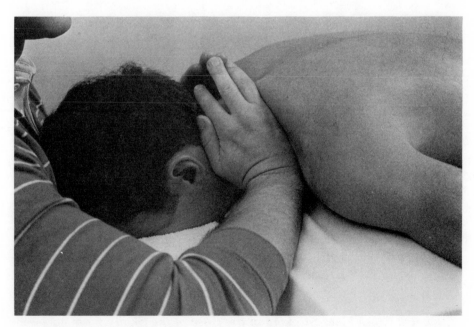

Blading of the Trapezius Placing the sides of the hands on either side of the neck, push down and out, maintaining pressure on the entire length of the trapezius. Repeat at least three times.

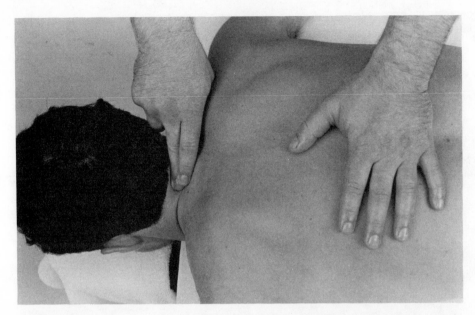

Local Cross-Fiber Stroking Between the Vertebrae From beside the
athlete, place your lower hand on the back for stability and apply strokes to
the muscles between the seven neck vertebrae. Begin gently, covering the
space between each vertebra for several seconds before going on to the next
one. Repeat, pressing harder each time. Cover the area from the base of the
skull to the top of the shoulders at least three times.

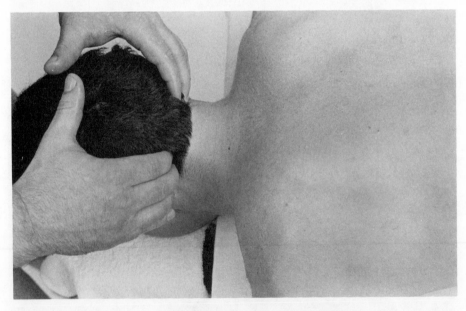

Local Cross-Fiber Stroking of the Base of the Skull From above the
athlete's head, administer local cross-fiber strokes to the base of the skull with
your fingertips. Cover the area all the way around the skull to just before the
ears. Repeat at least three times, probing as deeply as possible.

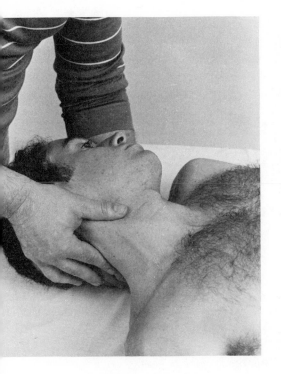

Broad Cross-Fiber Stroking of the Side of the Neck (Sternocleidomastoid) With the athlete on his back, assume a position above his head. Cradling the head with the palm of one hand, turn the head so the muscle running down the side of the neck is prominent. With thumb and fingers, stroke across the muscle from the ear to the base of the neck. Repeat this at least three times.

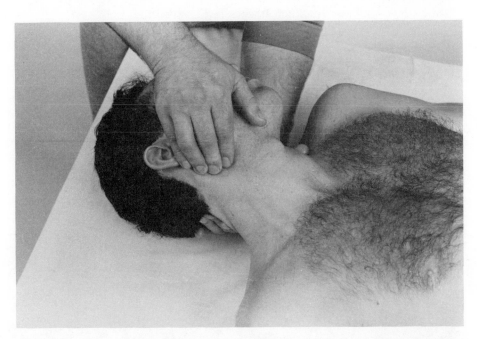

Local Cross-Fiber Stroking of the Side of the Neck Maintaining the athlete's head in the turned position, move to the side and administer local cross-fiber strokes to the muscle on the side of the neck, performing the movement from the ear to the base of the neck. Repeat at least three times.

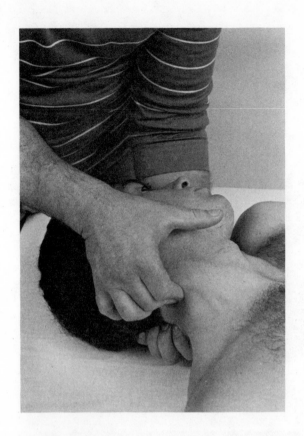

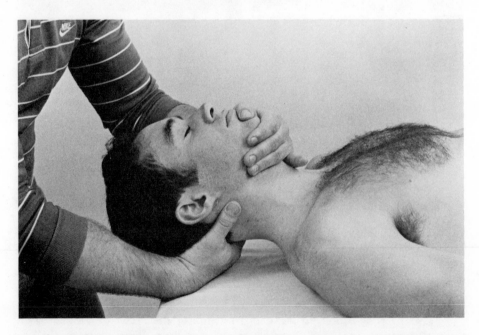

***Local Cross-Fiber Stroking and Stretching of the Muscles Adjacent to
the Cervical Spine (Semispinalis and Splenius Capitis)*** Cradling the athlete's head in the palm of one hand, use your fingertips to administer local

cross-fiber strokes to the muscles at the base of the skull. Apply cross-fiber strokes for one minute, then perform a neck stretch, pulling on the neck with the free hand placed beneath the athlete's chin. Pull for approximately thirty seconds and repeat the procedure: local cross-fiber strokes first, followed by the neck pull. Repeat three times on each side of the neck.

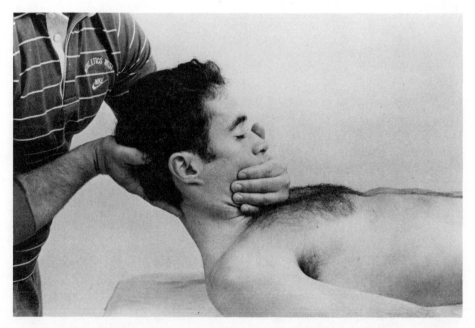

Neck Rotation   With one hand under the athlete's head and the other wrapped around his chin, raise the head slowly, bending the chin toward the chest. Hold for at least fifteen seconds before lowering the head. Repeat three times.